GDNF

What Happened To Me

GDNF

What Happened To Me

Stand Up, Shout Out, Be Counted

By

Andy Rollin

Cover image by Andy Rollin

Depicting the external port of the drug
delivery system which was implanted
within my head.

ISBN: 9798639239007

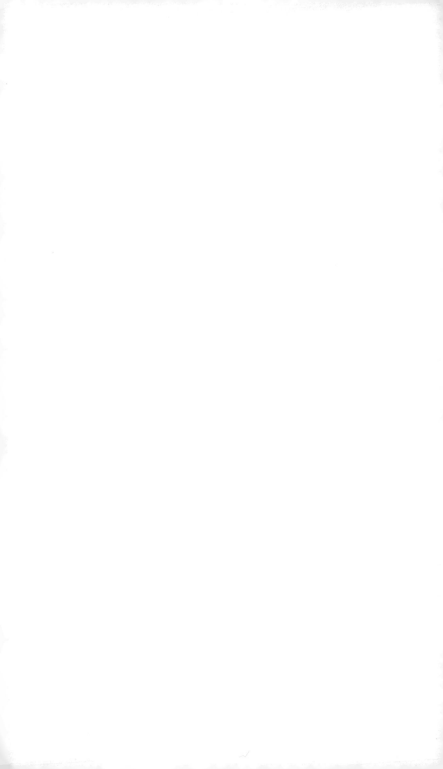

DEDICATION

To all the people with Parkinson's

that GDNF should be helping.

A SPECIAL THANK YOU TO

Anna, my childhood sweetheart, wife and understanding dance partner, I love you.

Chris and Sophie for being the wonderful people you are.

My Mum and Dad for always being there.

My family and friends for your love and support throughout the years.

Jayne and Darren, you are Batman and Robin to my Commissioner Gordon*.

All my proof readers whose positive comments gave me the confidence to proceed.

All the other GDNF'ers, I am lucky to know you.

All of the trial team for their respect, dignity, care and support, it was fun.

CONTENTS

*The use of * indicates an entry in the glossary*

INTRODUCTION

Parkinson's Disease is a progressive, degenerative, Neurological condition. There are over 145,000 people living with Parkinson's in the UK. Symptoms can include; involuntary shaking (known as tremor), slow movement, stiff and inflexible muscles, depression and anxiety, balance problems, loss of sense of smell, problems sleeping, memory problems and much more.

There is currently no cure and there have been no major advances in medication since the 1970's, with these treatments only masking the symptoms.

This account is based on my experiences before, during and after my participation in a clinical trial to discover if a naturally occurring protein called GDNF can slow, stop or even reverse Parkinson's.

GDNF was discovered in the 1990's and there have been several studies undertaken with varying results. GDNF's potential as a treatment for Parkinson's has been debated for many years and this was going to be the trial which would decide its future.

This trial, after many years of planning, started in 2013. Medgenesis, a Canadian Biotec company which owns the rights to GDNF, later announced a partnership with Pfizer to develop the drug.

My involvement began in March 2015. This is not a story, these events actually happened.

Before

Hello, my name is Andy Rollin. I live near Bristol with my wife Anna. We have two children, Chris and Sophie. Together with my brother I run a small family building business.

In June 2010, when I was aged 47, I was diagnosed with Parkinson's Disease. I had, of course, heard of it but surely only old people got it and they just shake a bit.

I had, over the previous 12–18 months, developed a shake in my right arm, which I had done nothing about. When I eventually went to my GP, he called it a 'tremor' and asked me to perform various arm movements.

Declaring 'At least it is not Parkinson's', he referred me to see a Neurologist at Frenchay Hospital.

A few weeks later, the Neurologist watched as I walked from the hospital waiting room into his surgery and sat me down.

He said. 'You have Parkinson's Disease.' He had spotted the classic symptoms; a lack of arm swing and tremor within a few seconds and arranged for me to have a DAT scan.

A DAT scan is a test to look at the level of dopamine receptor cells in the brain. It uses a small amount of an iodine based radioactive material. You lie on your back on a bed with your head in a small cradle while two cameras move around your head to create the images. The procedure takes around 30 minutes to complete.

This confirmed my diagnosis as there was a 'striking reduction in activity from the lentiform nuclei bilaterally'. My brain cells were dying.

I went home and continued with some decorating I was doing at the time. I knew nothing about Parkinson's and as they say, ignorance is bliss. I made no effort to learn about it.

I was then referred to Dr Alan Whone's 'Movement Disorders' clinic.

It was on a Saturday in late October 2010 that I had my first appointment with Dr Whone. He examined me and confirmed my diagnosis, we discussed the progression of Parkinson's.

He told me that 'there was typically very slow progress, particularly if you develop it at a young age and that he would be treating me for many decades to come.'

I was reassured and felt confident to be in his care. I quickly discovered that you should allow plenty of time when you have an appointment with Dr Whone as he did not have the timer running when you saw him. He gave every patient the time

5

needed to resolve any problems, be it 10 minutes or an hour. I did not mind waiting because I knew that when I needed extra time, I would receive it.

Gradually over the next few years, I settled into a routine of visiting Frenchay Hospital every 6–9 months to see Dr Whone. Medications were added, removed and adjusted in order to try and improve my symptoms. Sadly, most visits resulted in more medication.

I struggled with the fatigue and tremor whilst still working full time doing a physical job. Slowly other symptoms started to appear; loss of sense of taste and smell, my hand writing became smaller and smaller until it was so small, even I could not read it. Loss of dexterity in my hands meant I found it difficult to pick up small items.

The tremor made typing a lengthy exercise, with constant repetition of the same letter or number which I would then have to correct. I could not use a computer mouse without the spasms of my arm sending it haywire. I began to shuffle. The thing with Parkinson's is that it creeps up on you and you don't realise how much you've deteriorated until it's too late.

Night time was perhaps the worse time for me. After a day at work I was exhausted and needed a full night's sleep. Moving around in bed had become difficult. Whilst asleep I would remain perfectly still, not moving at all, which caused my back to seize up and become painful. The pain would then wake me after 3 maybe 4 hours of sleep, no need for an alarm clock. You would think that would satisfy Mr Parkinson's, but no. I then had to get out of bed which due to my rigid, contorted and painful body was a slow process.

I began by slowly easing myself to the edge of the bed then leaning against the head board and pushing until I was in a sitting position. This would take 2–3 minutes, all the time with my back throbbing. Once in a sitting position I then had to stand up, again slowly. Upon standing I then had to persuade my feet to move. Starting with a slow shuffle and gradually improving, until after 10–15 minutes, the pain and rigidity had eased and I could take my medication. This would take an hour or so to kick in, only then could normal service be resumed.

Life continued.

One evening in October 2013, we were watching the local news on TV when it was announced that there was to be a medical trial to see if something called GDNF could 'Slow, Stop or Reverse' the progression of Parkinson's. Dr Whone, as Chief Investigator, was being interviewed asking for people with Parkinson's to apply.

I was interested and visited the Parkinson's UK website to see what would be involved. You needed time off work, to undergo brain surgery and to attend monthly appointments at the hospital. I looked at the criteria and was secretly relieved to discover that you needed to have been diagnosed a minimum of 5 years.

I thought. 'that's OK, it has only been just over 4 years since I was diagnosed. I cannot apply'.

The following March I had my regular Outpatient's appointment with Dr Whone and I mentioned seeing him on TV. We had a chat about involvement in the trial and the commitment needed.

He asked 'Would you like to apply?'

I hesitated; he could see that I wasn't sure.

Then he said 'Maybe you would like to wait for the next one.'

Again, I had found a good reason not to apply. We went home and I started to regret my decision almost immediately.

I spent nearly a year disappointed in myself for not applying and wondering what might have been. One evening I was browsing the Parkinson's UK website, when I came across an article on the trial saying that they were still looking for participants. I had already made my decision over the previous few months; I was going to apply.

Without any discussion or consultation, I announced to all my family and friends that I was going to apply for the trial. Everyone was really positive about my decision, who knows what they are really thinking, particularly Anna. As a nurse she could foresee the pitfalls I was unaware of and, although very supportive, was extremely worried. With good reason. After all it was only experimental brain surgery, followed by having an experimental drug infused through an experimental delivery system. We had a young family and a mortgage to pay. I was being reckless in the extreme. Not only with my life, but with my family's life style, for that I apologise.

On the 4th of March 2015 I applied through the Parkinson's UK website and waited. Two days later while at work on a rooftop I receive a phone call from the trial administrator, Hannah. We talked for several minutes with her going through my application form with me, asking about my 'on' and 'off' periods.

'What is an 'on' or 'off' period' I thought to myself. I was to discover that I had been having 'off' periods for a long time, but thought it was extreme fatigue.

My knowledge of Parkinson's really was non-existent. I went to the hospital maybe twice a year and took whatever medication I was given. We ended the call

by arranging a visit to the trial team at
Monks Park House at Southmead Hospital,
for a chat about the trial and an initial
assessment on the following Wednesday.

THE ASSESSMENTS

My appointment is scheduled for 9.00 a.m. on Wednesday the 11th March 2015, I am going with Anna. It was going to prove very useful having a wife who, being a nurse, has a staff parking permit.

They say there are seven wonders in this world, meeting Anna and having our children count as my seven, but I was about to find number eight*. We say our goodbyes and go our different ways, Anna to work and me to one of the most extraordinary, positive and rewarding periods of my life, via Monks Park House.

I am greeted in the waiting room by Lucy, the senior research nurse, and we spend an hour or so together. She explains to me in great detail what would be happening during the trial or more correctly 'A Placebo-Controlled, Randomised, Double-

Blind trial to Assess the Safety and Efficacy of Intermittent Bilateral Intraputamenal Glial Cell Line-Derived Neurotrophic Factor (GDNF) Infusions Administered via Convection Enhanced Delivery (CED) in Subjects with Parkinson's Disease'.

It is in fact two separate trials, the first a Placebo-Controlled, Randomised, Double-blind trial for 40 weeks.

Infusions would happen every four weeks with off-medication assessments every eight week. Various scans, blood and cognitive tests would be done throughout. This is the gold standard trial where no one, doctors or participants, would know who is receiving the GDNF or Placebo. This is to help prevent the 'Placebo Effect' where by participants improve because they think they are receiving a new treatment even if they are not. It is very important that trials followed this design or the scientific community would not accept the results.

14

Secondly the 'Extension Trial', again, 40 weeks in duration with the same infusions, assessments, scans and tests. The big difference being that it was to be 'open label' where all the participants would receive GDNF.

There was a video to watch explaining the difference in relationship between a researcher and participant compared with a doctor and patient. I answer a short questionnaire and then Lucy shows me the layout of the delivery system and where it would be fitted on my head, with the help of a mannequin called Mike. He doesn't say much but I think he was a bit annoyed in case I take his place on the trial. He is, however, very good at illustrating where all the 'plumbing' was going to be fitted but not how it was going to be installed.

Lucy continued, saying 'The trial is being filmed for a BBC documentary.'

She asks 'Would you like to be involved?'

I declined; it is not really my cup of tea. I am quite a private person and the idea of being the centre of attention and on telly fills me with dread. I think of being followed around for days on end and say 'Definitely not.'

We have a short refreshment break and then I am to see Dr Whone. The doctor is his usual charming self and sets about running through what the trial involves in minute detail. His very relaxed manner immediately fills me with confidence and confirms in my mind that what I am doing is the right thing.

He is concerned about how the time commitment will affect my business. I had spoken about this with my brother and we had decided to play the long game. Sacrificing the time I would need for my recovery, in addition to the monthly visits against the hope that I may be able to carry on working to a normal retirement age, if the treatment proves to be successful.

We move on to what the surgery would involve. Basically, an incision across the top of my head with the skin being peeled back. 4 holes would then be drilled through my skull and 4 tubes inserted through my brain until they reach the area affected by the Parkinson's. These tubes would then be placed under the skin and connected to a port positioned behind my ear. Once every 4 weeks I would have an infusion of either Placebo or GDNF, a growth protein which should act like Baby Bio* and help to regrow brain cells. He tells me to expect nothing but to hope for an improvement, there are to be no guarantees.

He explains all of the risks and then tells me. 'You could end up worse than now, if that happens, we will try to repair any damage, but again there are no guarantees.'

17

He gives me a brief history of GDNF.
Telling me that Professor Steven Gill had
carried out a successful trial using pumps
situated within the abdomen at Frenchay
Hospital. He also mentioned that an
American trial had been stopped early due
to safety concerns and that the
participants had taken unsuccessful legal
action to try to receive ongoing infusions.
There were no guarantees that I would
continue to receive GDNF after the trial
had finished.

He asks what my family thought, so I tell
him that everyone was being very
supportive. However, Anna did not really
want me to do it. She was worried that
something horrible might happen. My son,
Chris, is like Anna and can see only the
possible problems. My daughter, Sophie,
who is younger and more gung-ho than
any of us said 'Go for it.'

He announces 'You meet all the criteria for
the trial, subject to passing all of the

assessments would you like to participate?'

I readily agreed and we sign the consent form. He tells me 'The trial is nearly closing and things will be moving fast.'

We make an appointment for the day after tomorrow Friday the 13th of March for the next assessment.

On Friday, I arrive at the hospital in good time for my 12.30 p.m. appointment and make my way to Monks Park House. As I wait, I hope that I will pass the assessments that would then allow me to become part of the trial. I sit quietly reading my book when a nurse comes into the room and calls my name. As I follow her down the corridor, I notice how 'hotch potch' the clinic area is with a definite make do and mend atmosphere.

The trial had recently moved from Frenchay Hospital, which was closing, and they are waiting to move into Elgar House.

Part of which will become 'The Bristol Brain Centre' a joint venture between the North Bristol NHS Trust and the University of Bristol to create a facility for clinical research teams to investigate Neurological diseases. But in the meantime, the trial team has to rough it in Monks Park House.

We enter one of the side rooms which is set up as a surgery and sit around a desk. The nurse introduces herself as Marisa and one of the trial doctors, Jack. She asks me questions about having Parkinson's, my general health and what medications I take. We then move onto a memory and thinking test, which is surprisingly difficult. I complete some questionnaires about my mood and Marisa assesses me for impulsive and compulsive behaviour. This is a major side effect of some of the Parkinson's medication.

I tell her 'Anna thinks my collection of books is getting to be compulsive' and add that I thought 'There was a fine line between being a collector and having a compulsion, and although I can and do control my purchases. I enjoy seeing my books lined up on the shelf.'

We agree that I am a collector not a compulsive.

We move onto the smell test. This is a booklet which has different smells, like grass, petrol and so on, impregnated onto each page which you activate by rubbing a pencil on it. I am shocked by the small number of smells that I can detect at all.

It is another example of how Parkinson's creeps up on you. It reminds me of when I used to suffer with hay fever from the age of around 15 until my mid-30's and then it just stopped. Was this an early sign of my Parkinson's starting to take over, slowly destroying the sensitivity of my nasal passages?

Jack takes over to perform a short physical examination. An ECG*, my first but by no means last, he measures my blood pressure which is slightly high but he puts this down to white coat syndrome*. I am given diaries for 3 days, to complete before I return, these will record the severity of my Parkinson's.

Dr Whone and Lucy then pop in to see me explaining that 'today has been successful and if convenient, there is a slot available for me to have the surgery on the 24th of March. Assuming that I pass the off-medication assessment.'

'That is only 10 days away.' I say to myself, while at the same time agreeing to do it.

This means having to squeeze the pre-trial off-medication assessment and the mapping scan into just over a week. I am given an appointment for Wednesday the 18th of March to continue the process.

On the day before the assessment I have a phone call cancelling it. The nurse who was performing it is ill. The appointment is rearranged for the Thursday instead and Dr Whone will be carrying it out. This, of course, has the knock-on effect of pushing the surgery back.

I don't take my slow release medication on the Wednesday morning and take my last dose of Carbidopa/levodopa at 6.00p.m. that evening. This ensures that all of my Parkinson's medication will out of my system by Thursday morning.

The off-medication assessment is going to be filmed so I need to be at Medical Illustrations Gate 38 for an 8.30 a.m. start. As there is a maze of roadworks on our route. We plan to leave at 7.00 a.m., with a possible journey time of up to an hour, to travel the 7 miles to our destination, the staff car park. Which has been temporally relocated to the BAWA* car park on Southmead Road during the re-building of the hospital, which should leave an easy 10-minute walk to the hospital.

When I wake, I realise what being off-medication actually means. This is the first time since my diagnosis that I have been without medication and I don't like it. Without realising it, I have become old and infirm, with the pills hiding the truth from me. I am 53 and am feeling like 93. Overnight I have developed a stoop, I am dragging my feet and shuffling along like an old man. How are we going to cope? How much longer can I work?

We set off with Anna driving because I am off-medication and arrive in good time. As we set off from the car park. I realise that we will not be rushing, I am finding it difficult to put one foot in front of the other. I am tired already and Anna, who only has little legs and usually meanders slowly along, keeps having to stop and wait for me to catch her up. I'm on the lookout in case Jeremy Beadle* emerges from behind a bush to tell me it has all been a joke and I can walk normally, but he doesn't.

As we reach the hospital entrance I am really flagging, we run into Dr Whone who is hurrying along carrying a large pile of files. He is on his way to my assessment and is dropping the files off somewhere on the way. He stops to talk to us and expresses his concern about me.

He asks 'Can you manage?'

I want to get there under my own steam so we carry on along the full length of the atrium, nearly 300m, and up to the top floor. Eventually arriving at Medical Illustrations.

We are greeted by Andrew who, it turns out, will film all of my assessments throughout the trial. Anna leaves to go to work and Dr Whone arrives shortly afterwards. He greets me and asks 'How are you feeling?'

So, I reply 'I am grateful you are taking such good care of me.'

I explain that normally I feel so much better than this, and am only now realising how much I rely on my medication.

We walk into the assessment room; I later find out that some participants refer to it as 'The Torture Chamber.' It is really a film studio fully equipped with lighting and so on. The assessments are being carried out to obtain my UPDRS score or Unified Parkinson's Disease Rating Scale score. This is a rating system accepted by the scientific community upon which the success or failure of the trial will be based. It's out of 100, the higher the score the more severe the Parkinson's. The assessments will involve testing my levels of stiffness, speed of hand movements and walking ability.

We begin with Dr Whone showing me a series of hand movements which I have to repeat as many times as possible during a timed period. This is followed by; timed finger taps, assessment of body rigidity, a vocal assessment, an assessment of how well I can recover after being pulled backwards sharply and a timed walk. This marks the end of the 'off' medication part and Dr Whone gives me double my usual dose of Carbidopa/levodopa. This is an attempt at returning me to a fully 'on' state, which will be necessary to carry on with the assessments.

We leave the assessment room; a cup of tea is made for me and I rest for around about an hour reading my book. Being 'off' feels like you are in a dark and dingy room, the curtains are shut, you have candyfloss in your ears and you are standing in a bucket of concrete.

Slowly I return to my normal drugged state; movement becomes easier and my head begins to clear, first the candyfloss disappears and then the curtains are opened and finally I step out of the bucket. Once I have fully recovered, we return to the assessment room and repeat the assessment in a fully 'on' condition.

All of this has taken around three hours. Dr Whone and I return to Monks Park House; where he gives me more questionnaires concerning quality of life to complete. I hand in the diaries I had been given previously. Anna joins me, and both of us then have a long talk about the trial with Dr Whone. He answers any questions or concerns we have; I am then offered a place on the trial which I gratefully accept. We turn our attention to the Mapping scan this needs to be carried out quickly He checks the available dates and arranges it for the 25th of March to be followed by surgery on the 2nd of April. This will be just before Easter which is fine after all what could possibly go wrong?

Mapping scan and surgery

The Mapping scan is probably one of the most important procedures that is going to be carried out. On a very basic level, it shows details of your brain slice by slice all the way through. This will enable the surgical team to plan the best route through the brain to the target area with pin point accuracy, missing all the important bits like blood vessels and so on.

It's an MRI scan, however, as accuracy is so important, it is performed under a general anaesthetic as the patient has to remain completely still for the entire duration. Once asleep, a 'reference frame' is fitted to the head, think 'The Man in the Iron Mask*' updated and crossed with Hannibal Lector*. There are location points on the frame which fit into the ears and once it's correctly positioned there are bolts that are tightened against the skull to secure it. Not very pretty, but invaluable as a guide to the correct alignment of the tubes.

On Wednesday the 25th of March, Anna and I arrive at Gate 20 for the mapping scan. We are waiting in a side room when the door is opened by a man in scrubs who introduces himself as Christian, Steven Gill's registrar, we discuss the procedure.

He tells us that 'a slot has opened up to carry out the surgery on Saturday.'

This is only 3 days away, although I am surprised at the speed things are happening.

I agree. 'It will be fine.'

At this point I don't want to wait any longer. The conversation moves on to the positioning of the port and what is likely to happen on Saturday. Christian leaves and I am ushered through into a waiting area with several trolleys dotted around. Anna has to wait in the main waiting room, but I think she will disappear for a coffee, or more likely a hot chocolate with all the trimmings.

I am soon joined by an anaesthetist who goes through all the paperwork with me. We then start chatting about the success the trial already seems to be.

He puts a cannula into the back of my hand and asks me to lie down, he injects a solution into the cannula.

Saying 'You will feel sleepily……'

Then I am awake, it is a couple of hours later and I am in the recovery area with a nurse calling out my name. It has all been done while I was sleeping. Anna enters the room and everything is OK. I have a cup of tea, and over the course of an hour or so I gradually return to normal and the staff are happy for me to go home. Anna is sent to bring the car around to the main hospital entrance, being told to 'ignore the parking Nazi's, if they try to move you on.'

We give Anna a head start,
and then the nurse pushes me in a wheelchair down through the atrium to where Anna is waiting outside.

Saturday the 28th of March, surgery day. We wake early as we have to be back at Gate 20 for 7.30 a.m., nothing to eat as I am scheduled to be in surgery around 10.00 a.m. I drive, both to stop me thinking too much and because after today I will not be able to drive for four weeks. My mind wanders and I start counting the days, is it only 22 days since that phone call from Hannah while I was at work? I marvel at how things have changed in that short space of time. I park the car and give the keys to Anna, after all I will not be needing them for a while.

As we arrive at Gate 20, we are taken straight through to the Medi-rooms. The nurse tells us that the surgical team are having a meeting to discuss the running order. Apparently, there is another participant having his surgery today as well.

The anaesthetist arrives shortly after and proceeds to update us, I am to go down second probably about 1.00 p.m. He suggests that we 'go walkabout'* as long as I do not eat or drink anything. So, Anna and I slowly meander down to the atrium to ring the family who, by now, were expecting me to be on the table.

We read our books instead of talking about the day's events, wander around the grounds and gently make our way back to the medi-rooms by noon and are greeted with the news that things are progressing well and I should start to get ready.

I am given a gown which ties up at the back, so I am grateful for Anna's help in attempting to preserve my modesty, but it's still a bit draughty. Next come the surgical stockings, they are different from my usual kind, but will help to reduce the risk of blood clots. There is no way I can put them on by myself. Anna offers to help, but after 20 minutes struggling with them, I am grateful when the nurse returns and seeing the trouble, we are having she takes over and has the stockings on in a couple of minutes. Her secret is to put my foot into the bag the stockings have come in, this allows the tight tube to easily slide onto my leg with the bag being removed afterwards in a second. She then proceeds to put a cannula into the back of my hand and we are ready for action.

I'm all dressed up with nowhere to go, so we wait, trying to make small talk without mentioning what is about to happen. At

3.30 p.m. the door opens and Christian walks in, they are ready for me. Anna dissolves into tears, we have a cuddle, kiss and say our goodbyes. Then we walk along the corridor with Christian leading the way, we turn a corner and Anna is gone. Christian holds a door open for me and I walk directly into the operating theatre. I stop and look around; it is like being on the bridge of the Star Ship Enterprise*. All the equipment, tiny lights flashing everywhere, I expect to see Captain Kirk* striding through the doors demanding 'More thrust Scotty*.'

There is a window through which I can see the staff washing their hands. On the left are several light boxes covered in scans of my head, alongside that is the robot which will be used to align the tubes. In the middle is the operating table with Steven Gill standing beside it. He introduces himself, and we have a very brief chat.

He tells me. 'You are the penultimate person to have the surgery.' and jokes 'Hopefully we've got things right now.'

He moves away to talk to someone, and the anaesthetist appears, as if by magic, just like Mr Benn*!

He is talking to me and at the same time filling the cannula.

He asks me 'To count......'

I don't know what number I get to …… and then I am waking up, a nurse calling my name. I am back in the medi-rooms, somewhere between sitting up and lying down, slowly I am coming around.

The nurse is telling me 'Your wife has been ringing to see how you are and is on her way in.'

I ask 'What is the time?'

'11.00 p.m.' Is the reply.

That means I have been asleep seven hours at least; Anna must have been going out of her mind with worry. A porter arrives and I am taken to the Neurological ward, Anna and Sophie, our daughter, are both there waiting. It is really good to see them, they gingerly hug me and then they are being gently moved back out of the door.

Anna says 'We will be back in the morning.'

The staff set about making me comfortable, giving me my medication, which is hopelessly late and making me a cup of tea which is greatly appreciated as my throat is so dry. I need to use the toilet.

I ask 'Can I get out of bed?'

The nurse returns with a disposable bottle which I know that no matter how desperate I am I cannot use. Reluctantly he agrees and I ease myself out of bed and shuffle into the shower room. Mission accomplished! I turn and look in the mirror. It is still me, wearing the by now crumpled gown and on my head is a tightly bound bandage resembling a large white turban. I return to bed and sleep half sitting up only being disturbed when the nurse comes in to check on me.

I awake slightly before 6.00 a.m., lying still on the bed. I ponder upon the things that have happened and things that are yet to come, quietly coming to until I am fully awake. The nurse eases her head around the door.

'Morning' I say.

She comes into the room, surprised to see me awake, she records my observations and dispenses my usual medication.

I ask 'Can I get up?'

She agrees. 'That should be fine.'

I use the facilities, change out of the gown and into the specially purchased pyjamas and put on my dressing gown. Instead of returning to bed, I move the chair next to the window and watch all the people hurrying past on their way to work whilst texting my brother to update him, who says men cannot multi-task.

I ask him 'Can you pass the message onto mother?'

Mother, like most parents, worries about us constantly. If we travel more than 20 miles, she likes us to ring so she knows we are OK. But conversely, she has a mobile phone which is never turned on, as 'it's only for emergencies' so if we need to contact her, we never can.

He replies within a few moments, surprised that I am up and around. I have also texted Anna but she doesn't reply until later as she only checks her phone every couple of days.

Breakfast is served, toast and tea. I read my book and two health care assistants arrive to help me wash and dress. I am already up so they leave me to my book.

Around 10.30 a.m. Christian and some of the surgical team arrive to check on me. They are pleased that I am up and about.

They ask 'How are you feeling? Do you have any pain?'

I reply 'Absolutely fine, no pain at all.'

Apparently tomorrow, Monday, I will be having the bandage removed and then on Tuesday I can go home.

Everything is going nicely to plan, no problems or hiccups. Anna and Sophie turn up just as the others are leaving bringing cups of hot chocolate and nervous smiles.

Anna is looking at me as if she is running through an inventory in her mind. Two legs, check, two arms, check, one head, check. All present and accounted for, she smiles.

I ask how she had filled the time yesterday afternoon. She explains that she had wanted to stay until I came out, but the nurses had persuaded her to go home. Where she spent the time pacing around the house looking for things to do, unable to concentrate on anything and periodical bursting into tears.

Eventually by 7.00 p.m. she could wait no longer and rang the hospital, only to be told that I was still in theatre. They should be finished by now, the doubt then joined with the worry.

Sophie tells me. 'Mum was in pieces.'

After several phone calls Anna hears the words she has been waiting for, I was out of theatre. By now it was nearly 11.00 p.m., and she told the nurse they were on their way in.

I hug Anna, trying to reassure her but failing dismally. We spend a happy afternoon chatting, reading and with Sophie making fun of my 'turban'. Chris will not be visiting as he has a bad cold and anyway, I am coming home on Tuesday.

Monday arrives I am up reading from 6.00 a.m. again. Around 10.30 a.m. the nurse comes into the room.

And asks 'Shall we remove the bandage?'

She sits me in a chair and standing behind me begins unwinding the coils from around my head it seems to be endless as my head is slowly revealed.

I ask 'What does it look like?'

She replies 'Fine' and fetches a mirror so I can take a look, but no matter how we position it I cannot see a thing. I go into the shower room and look in the mirror, nothing. All I can see is my blood clogged hair. Anna looks later and says 'Ummm.'

Then gets out her phone and takes a few pictures, at first, I cannot make out what I am looking at. I look again, my hair is a bloody mess and in the middle is a reddish disc with a piece of yellow stained gauze surrounding it, resembling a vampire's eye after a blood-soaked orgy.

Later in the afternoon I am asked by the nurse 'Seeing as you will be going home tomorrow do you mind moving to the Procedure Room?'

When the hospital was being planned, it was decided that it would be nice to have a room on every ward where small medical procedures could be carried out without the patient having to leave the ward 'The Procedure Room'. Of course, in reality it is never used for this, doubling up as a spare bed space come storage room. Which usually houses a selection of spare chairs, equipment and maybe a desk as well. A bed has been squeezed into one corner with a small table alongside it. On top of this table a small hand bell has been placed in order to summon help if required. A token gesture really, as there is no way that the bell would be heard on a busy ward. There is only a small window instead of a floor to ceiling, wall to wall panoramic window in the standard rooms.

The toilet facilities are located along the ward corridor, in an extremely large room into which beds can be wheeled and patients washed in-situ. The toilet is positioned against the far wall approximately 20 feet from the door, which is locked with one of those locks that can be opened from outside, with only a coloured indicator to protect against an interruption.

 I agree after all I am going home in the morning.

AFTERMATH IN THE DOLDRUMS

I wake on Tuesday morning, as usual, just before 6.00 a.m. again. I am in the Procedure Room, there is a desk in front of the window, so no sitting by it to view the outside world. I will have to sit on the bed to read while I wait to go home, never mind it is only going to be for a few hours. I get up, wash and dress. And I wait, the other thing about being in the Procedure Room is you tend to get forgotten. Eventually the nurse comes in and starts to do my observations, she does them again.

She asks 'Do you feel alright?'

'Yes' I reply 'Why?'

Apparently, my heart rate is 167, she leaves the room and quickly returns with the on-call doctor. A young junior doctor nearing the end of a long night shift, who has just been told that one of the patients may have a heart problem. She confirms my heart rate and then leaves to get some assistance. When she returns, she is in the company of another slightly more senior doctor, he explains that I have an extremely high heart rate and that they have asked one of the Cardiologists to come and have a look at me. In the meantime, he asks the junior doctor to put a cannula in to save time later.

It does not look like I will be going home today.

She is clearly in a bit of a panic as she goes about attempting to insert the cannula. No matter what she does she cannot find a vein, we end up with a mass of tape all over the back of my hand and instead of lying flat on my hand the cannula sticks up at a funny angle.

She leaves and when the nurse returns, she looks at my hand and says 'I think we had better do that again, shall we?'

The senior doctor returns with the Cardiologist. He says that 'Such a high heart rate is dangerous and that they are going to try and lower it.'

He asks me to 'Hold my breath, this will increase the pressure in my belly which should bring the heart rate down.'

It does not.

'OK we will do a Chemical Cardioversion.' He says and explains that they will chemically interrupt the heart rhythm which will allow the heart to reset itself. A bit like rebooting a computer.

They are going to stop my heart.

I will have to be moved to a cardiac ward for it to be carried out, I agree and ring Anna to tell her what is about to happen and that I am moving. Shortly after I am transferred to a cardiac ward on a four bedded bay. The Cardiologist and the Neurologist are preparing for the procedure and are talking to each other.

The Neurologist says. 'I have never done this before.'

To which the Cardiologist replies 'It's OK I've done it a couple of times.'

I am filled with confidence. I appreciate that the only way to learn is to have a go, but I would prefer if they were not practising on me.

At this point Anna arrives and hurries over to us. Spotting the resus* trolley positioned close by she starts to well up. After all she has just rushed to the hospital after being told that I have a problem with my heart and have been moved to a cardiac ward and the first thing she sees upon arrival is the resus* trolley next to me.

The Cardiologist jumps up to reassure her that it is only a precaution, just in case. The procedure starts. I am warned that I will feel a strange sensation, starting in my legs which will rise through my body until it reaches my head, when it will disappear. The Cardiologist gives the Neurologist a syringe filled with a 'flushing' solution.

And tells him 'To flush the cannula through when I say so.'

The Cardiologist administers the drug through the cannula and I wait for the promised sensation. Something is happening, I can feel it in my feet, which builds in intensity, it is weird but not horrific and it passes over so quickly it hardly registers.

'NOW!' The Cardiologist shouts.

The cannula is flushed through and my heart rate is checked, no change, as before, the procedure has not worked.

'Oh' says the disappointed Cardiologist 'We had better not do that again.'

My faith in their ability soars.

There are no spare rooms on the cardiac ward so I am going to be moved back to another Neurological ward. While I am waiting for the porter, lunch is being served to the other patients; I'm just visiting so nothing for me. There are raised voices on the other side of the ward. Apparently a newly admitted patient is being given what his predecessor had ordered and is not pleased, 'a ham sandwich, but hold the ham.'

The porter arrives and I am moved. I wait all day for a Cardiologist to come and review me but no one arrives, I will be seen tomorrow.

It is now Wednesday the 1st of April 2015, very apt. I am still waiting to see a Cardiologist; the day passes slowly, I am on a Neurology ward but my Neurological treatment has finished, I am in the way, bed blocking. Mid-afternoon I am asked if I will move to the Procedure Room again because they desperately need the bed.

Thinking that the doctor will be arriving soon I agree again, on condition that once I have seen the doctor, they will find me a room if I need to stay in. I move to the procedure room but I still do not see a doctor. Lucy and Jack, the trial doctor, come to see me and express surprise that I am still waiting to see a Cardiologist.

Thursday, I wait in the Procedure Room all day, going a bit stir crazy. A medical student pops her head around the door and asks 'Would you mind answering a few questions as part of some research I am doing?'

I virtually drag her in desperate for a diversion to the tedium. I then proceed to bore her rigid about why I am in hospital and the trial before she can escape. Still no doctor, it's like I am in 'The Twilight Zone*'. Jack pops in early evening, he is on his way home and asks 'Have you been seen by a doctor?'

He is angry with the answer saying 'Leave it with me.'

An hour later Jack returns, he has not gone home, he has been trying to contact a cardiologist.

He tells me 'One of the cardiologists will come to review you tomorrow after they have completed their own ward round.'

I thank him.

It's Good Friday, not that it makes any difference to me. Just before lunch a lady cardiologist knocks on the door, thanks to Jack.

I have been waiting four days to be reviewed, she explains that as soon as there is a room available on the Cardiology ward, I will be moved. Unfortunately, it is going to be a few days. This must be how Joseph felt, I think about asking her if we are in Bethlehem not Southmead*, she leaves. I remind the nurses of their promise, reluctantly I am moved to a proper room, it's great and I settle in.

Two hours later a nurse comes into the room, I think she has come to take my blood pressure or something but, no.

She asks me 'Would you mind moving to the Procedure Room?'

I refuse.

She says something about 'Clinical need.'

I tell her 'To get security if you want to move me.'

I am not very popular.

Saturday, it's the Easter weekend, everything seems to have stopped. Chris is better so he visits, I have missed him.

Easter Sunday I am moving to a cardiac ward at last, I gather my things together and wait, just after lunch it happens. We arrive at the ward and I am pushed into a 4 bedded bay, my worst nightmare. It is very busy with visitors; Anna stays until teatime.

Things become more settled as people leave, but there are several TV's loudly blaring out. An elderly gentleman in the opposite corner gets out of bed and strips off before he walks naked to the shower room being chased by a nurse. It seems like I've fallen through a black hole and emerged in 'The Benny Hill Show*.'

It's 9.00 p.m. and a nurse is handing out bottles to the patients, I refuse one. The lights are dimmed, I can hear the bottles being filled and patients getting in and out of bed. Eventually things slow down but the ward doors still bang as staff move about. Then the nurses start to discuss

54

where they are going next weekend, what they are going to do and to whom.

I hardly sleep and I am still lying awake at 5.00 a.m. when a nurse comes in to check on me, she sees that I am still awake.

'Are you OK?' she asks.

I reply. 'No.' Explaining why and request that, if possible, can I be moved to a single room soon.

Bob Geldof did not like Mondays*, but I do. I am moved to a single room but I have to wear a heart monitor 24 hours a day, the lead is just long enough to reach the toilet which is handy. After lunch Jack and a nurse arrive to remove my stitches as it has been nine days since my operation. They cause quite a stir amongst the staff as they sit me down and start. Jack examines the wound and comments on how well it's healing, which is good news.

Jack tells me to come over to Monks Park House when I am are discharged to collect some supplies for cleaning the wound.

They have only just gone when Marisa knocks on the door, she has come over to transcribe my hospital notes into my trial notes. She spots Anna and recognises her, it turns out they worked together at some point, small world as they say. I wake on Tuesday having slept much better, I have been prescribed some medication to lower my heart rate and it is working, the monitor is now showing 130, which is lower. By Thursday it is low enough and I am taken off the monitor and moved to a room further away from the nurse's station, must be a good sign.

Friday the 9th of April, it's our wedding anniversary, 27 years. We see the consultant and I can go home, in the words of the song 'I'm coming home I've done my time*'. Unfortunately, I have to wait for the pharmacy to sort out my medication and of course the bed is needed so I have to move to the discharge lounge.

When I arrive, I tell the nurse in charge 'I need to go over to Monks Park House to collect some supplies.'

She's not pleased and says 'You cannot go.'

I tell her 'I am going anyway you can accompany me if you like.'

Reluctantly she agrees and we wander over, as we sit waiting for Jack she's muttering under her breath.

So, I tell her 'Go and I will make my own way back.'

Just then Jack arrives with my bag of goodies, which I thank him for and we return to the discharge lounge. By the time we get back the pharmacy have delivered so we can go home. Brilliant. It is going to be another 4 weeks before I can return to work. That will fly by, Anna and I have booked a few days away in the Cotswolds, so we are looking forward to that.

TEST INFUSION AND PET SCAN

It is now the 27th of April 2015, a full month since my surgery and I have an appointment at Monks Park House at 8.30 a.m. It's an early start because it is a busy day, Anna drops me off, and I go into the waiting room and see another patient also waiting.

We are both called together so we introduce ourselves, his name is John and he is the person who had surgery on the same day as me. We are both escorted to Gate 19, MRI suite, for a scan to ensure that all is OK with the delivery system. I go in first, removing any metallic items beforehand. I lie on the table and I am given a pair of headphones to wear, my head is strapped into place to avoid movement. The table slides into the machine and the scan starts.

It is so loud, the machine clangs and bangs, the table moves in and out as they scan my brain. It only lasts 25 minutes but seems like forever, you have to lie perfectly still. Suddenly I am aware of people moving around the machine and the table slides out, it is over. I am helped to my feet and ushered out. John goes in.

I am asked to make my way promptly back to Monks Park House.

When I arrive, I am shown into the infusion room. This is where the magic is going to happen, a growth protein is going to be infused across the blood brain barrier, which has never been done before the trial started. A nurse greets me and introduces herself as Yolanda, it is her first day as well and she has brought in some chocolates which she passes around.

I am asked 'Do you need to use the toilet as you are going to be busy for a while, once we start, we cannot stop.'

I sit in a comfortable reclining chair and watch as they prepare for the test infusion that I will be receiving. The trial team will be infusing a placebo solution containing a dye which will show up on the MRI scan. This is to check that the delivery system is working properly and is capable of delivering GDNF to the correct area at sufficient strength. There appears to be yards and yards of very thin clear plastic tubing connecting the pumps to the port, all of which needs priming to ensure the flow is maintained.

Yolanda takes my blood pressure sitting and then standing, then records my temperature. Jack comes in saying that he has checked the MRI and there are no problems and he proceeds to make the final connection. On the end of all the tubing is a metal adaptor which links the tubing and pumps to my port. Jack makes the connection and tightens the retaining screw with a small screwdriver.

He then turns a wheel on the back of the adaptor which in turn pushes 4 metal needles through the silicone seal in my port and connects directly into the tubing buried within my head. The sensation, as the wheel is turned, can only be described as what it would feel like if you put your head into a pencil sharpener.

The pumps are turned on and I wait for the surge as the liquid is pumped into my brain, but nothing appears to happen. This is because the quantities being infused are tiny, similar in size to a tear drop, taking 1 hour and 40 minutes to complete. I settle down and read my book. Periodically my blood pressure is taken, the chair is comfortable and I begin to nod off.

Suddenly, the pumps are bleeping, apparently this is a warning that the infusion is nearly over, a couple more minutes and I am being disconnected.

I now need to be scanned again to check that the GDNF will be able to reach the target area. So, John and I return to Gate 19 to repeat the procedure. This time it seems quicker, easier, we finish and walk back to Monks Park House. As it was my first infusion, I will have to stay for another 3–4 hours to ensure I don't have any kind of reaction. By the time we get back, the MRI results have come through, this is important because if the target area does not have a certain amount of coverage, I could still be removed from the trial. Jack checks my results.

He declares 'This is probably the best spread I have seen.'

Its soon time to leave and I go to meet Anna and give her the good news.

Its now the 4th of June, a Thursday, it's been 6 weeks since my test infusion and I have heard nothing from the trial team. Everything seems to have ground to a halt, maybe they have lost my phone number. I feel slightly deflated after all the rush, rush, rush of the first month. Since my operation I have noticed people doing a double take when they spot the port on the side of my head. It is quite noticeable as my hair is short.

Anna says that 'It's getting thin.'

But I say 'It's not thin, I just chose to have it short.' There's a difference.

Anyway, people look quite obviously but they never say anything, which is a shame as I want to tell them all about it.

Today I have an Outpatient's appointment with Dr Whone. It was booked before I joined the trial and is in the main hospital building, perhaps I can get an update. I wait the usual hour or so past the appointment time and then it is my turn. This is the first time I have seen him since the off-medication assessment. He greets me warmly and wants to know every detail about my hospital stay. I also tell him about a recent appointment I had with my cardiac consultant. That I have got something called Atrial Fibrillation, which is an irregular heartbeat, the consultant thinks that I have probably always had it. It can be treated with medication and I am to have regular cardiac reviews. Dr Whone seems relieved that it was not caused by any of the trial treatment. I tell him that really, it was lucky that it happened now as we are aware of it and it can be monitored. Instead of finding out about by way of a cardiac incident later in life.

I think I was put on hold for the trial until the team were happy that it was safe for me to continue. Soon after seeing Dr Whone, I receive an appointment to have a PET scan for the 18th of June. Within days this appointment is cancelled due to a UK wide shortage of one of the drugs required to carry out the scan. The appointment is re-scheduled for Thursday the 9th of July, at the recently opened 'Bristol Brain Centre' for 9.30 a.m. The scan must be carried out off-medication, so no Parkinson's drugs, I am not looking forward to that.

On the day, Anna and I arrive early and sit in the waiting room. We are to travel to the University Hospital of Wales in Cardiff by taxi. I am off-medication and tired. Sue, one of the participants, accompanies us. She is waiting with Marisa, who is weighed down with all the medication and our hospital notes which she needs to take with her. We squeeze into the taxi and off we go.

Anna and Marisa start to reminisce about when they worked together, Sue and I, both off medication promptly fall asleep. 'On' periods are when your Parkinson's medication is working fully. 'Off' periods are when the medication doesn't work, these periods are generally unpredictable and can change very quickly.

The taxi drops us off outside the main entrance, Sue is being helped along by Marisa. Anna and I are bringing up the rear, Marisa keeps looking around asking 'Are you alright?'

She must have been here several times. Steering us through the crowds, navigating through a labyrinth of corridors and passageways with me following behind feeling like the minotaur* the day after a night down the pub.

We arrive at the department; Sue is first and goes straight in. The rest of us make ourselves comfortable. I read, Anna and Marisa resume their chat from where it was paused earlier. I am going in around 1.00 p.m., so at 11.45 a.m. we go for an early lunch. I have been off-medication since 6.00 p.m. yesterday and I am feeling it. When we return, I go straight in to be prepared.

The PET scan is going to be an important tool for the trial. By comparing subsequent scans, the team will be able to assess any restoration of the dopamine nerve endings in my brain.

First, a cannula is put into the back of my hand. Then a special dye containing radioactive tracers is injected via the cannula, these tracers can be detected by the scanner. I am then taken into the scanner, stopping on route at the toilet, at my age you never refuse the opportunity.

The scanner itself is similar to the MRI scanner in appearance and operation. Basically, a tube into which you are inserted with the machine moving around you taking pictures. I am surprised when the nurse settling me in asks if I could loosen my trousers. And brought back to reality when her colleague says 'No, we are doing the head.' Never mind.

I collapse onto the table and I am wedged in tight. By now I have been off-medication for nearly 20 hours and I know it. The scan is going to take an hour and a half, how can I stay perfectly still for so long? The scan starts, it's very loud. But I am like a caterpillar in my cocoon, nice and snug I close my eyes and fall into a deep sleep, I am so tired.

The next thing I know the table is moving out of the scanner and people are removing the padding. It is over, I collect myself and return to the waiting area where Anna and Marisa, now joined by an 'on medication 'Sue, are still putting the world to rights. At long last I can have my medication; I settle into the taxi and as I drift off to sleep wondering if global warming has been increased after all of Anna's efforts today. It has been a busy day.

THE TRIAL-066

Week 0

Tuesday the 14th of June 2015 is going to be my week 0, with my first off-medication assessment of the trial, again at Medical illustrations at 8.30 a.m. Anna escorts me directly there and then leaves for work. I sit in the small waiting area and am called by a nurse. Together, we walk along the corridor and into the assessment room. Andrew is ready and waiting for us so we exchange pleasantries 'nice to see you again and so on'.

The nurse tells me her name is Jeanette and her main role in the trial team is carrying out the assessments. Eventually she will carry out all of my assessments, we talk about life in general and discover we live in the same general area so we moan about how bad the traffic is.

We then begin the off-medication assessment. Her style is different from Dr Whone's, but we carry out the same exercises. She asks me to repeat a couple of things which I do not perform correctly. We get to the 'pulled backwards' part and she reassures me not to worry if I fall, she will catch me. I doubt this very much and think that Andrew may have to pick us both up. We finish and Jeanette gives me my double dose of medication and takes me to a waiting room, where she brings me a cup of tea. As I start to switch on, we complete some questionnaires about my abilities in an 'on' and 'off' state. On the top of the sheet is my name and a number; 066.

She explains '066 is your trial number and you are the last participant.'

I think, if my trial number is the last one and I was penultimate for the surgery, my start must have been delayed because of the complications. I get my book out to read while I fully switch on. Jeanette asks me. 'What book is it?'

We then proceed to chat about books as she is also a keen reader. We complete the 'on' assessment and return to the Brain Centre as there are more questionnaires to complete.

My next appointment is the following day in the Brain Centre at 9.30 a.m. I am shown into the newly refurbished infusion room. It is certainly a step up from Monks Park House.

This is to be my first proper infusion of either GDNF or Placebo and I am looking forward to starting. Yolanda is there as well as Jeanette There are also two new trial doctors Mihaela and Sonali. I ask after Jack, apparently, he has moved on. Already seated are two other participants who are being connected for infusions; Jeff and Lesley. We exchange only greetings as we have all been told not to

talk about the trial or anything connected
to it. This is annoying as it is all we want to
talk about. My seat is between the others
and after a short while Yolanda takes my
blood pressure. Apparently, it is high and
when she repeats it, the reading is still
high. She confers with Mihaela who comes
over, they retake the test together.
Mihaela disappears out of the infusion
room.

This is not a good start, given my recent
cardiac history and the fact that they
delayed my start to avoid this sort of event
happening. They probably have had a
meeting previously to decide if I should
continue and now this on my first infusion!

She returns about half an hour later with
Dr Whone, they draw the curtains around
me to give the illusion of privacy. They
have been to see my cardiac consultant
and discussed the development of high
blood pressure on top of my irregular
heart rhythm. They perform an ECG*

which is normal and they prescribe medication for my blood pressure. It is decided to carry on so I am connected and receive the infusion without incident. Again, I stay for 3 hours afterwards as a precaution.

It is a week after my infusion and I am experiencing something unusual. I can smell what can only be described as a strong solvent/metallic smell, it is everywhere but no one else can smell it.

Week 4

Wednesday the 12th of August, another infusion at the Brain Centre, no problems. I am getting the hang of this. My blood pressure is fine now I have started the new medication, everyone is a bit more relaxed today. I tell the team about the strange smell which faded after a few days and they note it as an adverse event.

Week 8

Today, the 9th of September, is the next off-medication assessment. It's a busy day as I'm also having an infusion. I do not feel too bad, Anna drives as usual and we park at BAWA*, I am not looking forward to the next part. We leave the car and start slowly down the road; Anna is mindful of the last time and is taking things slow. We have gone about 100 yards but I do not need to stop, I pick up the pace a bit, no problems. Anna realises that I am getting ahead of her and she speeds up but I continue to walk faster and faster, every step a tiny bit quicker.

Then I hear Anna's voice. 'Slow down, I can't keep up.'

I stop and wait for her, then we resume our journey at a brisk pace. I stride through the hospital grounds, continuing through the atrium into the lift and up to Medical Illustrations.

I cannot believe what has just happened, I am over the moon. The difference in my walking is astounding, I do not understand. I think back to that morning in March and go through what is different, nothing, except……. the two infusions I have received, that is all. I must be on the GDNF or is it the placebo effect we were warned about? No, it can't be, my imagination is not that good. If I am like this after two infusions what will I be like by the end of the trial? Am I cured?

She must see the smile on my face because Jeanette asks. 'Are you OK?'

I tell her of my 'Road to Damascus*' experience, she smiles but we cannot discuss it.

We perform the assessments, then I return to the Brain Centre and have an uneventful infusion. After being asked about adverse events, I tell the team about the improvement in my walking. Unfortunately, it is not noted as it would be qualitative evidence, which cannot be easily and accurately compared. The trial needs quantitative evidence which can be measured and compared with the other participants results.

I can't believe it; my experience must be of interest to someone.

The following week we are going away to Wales for a week. The first few days are uneventful, nice, happy days.

On the Wednesday I wake up, and without thinking about it, I sit up, swing my legs out of bed and stand up. I stand there pondering what is different. Is something wrong? Slowly the realisation of what has just happened sweeps over me. I have got out of bed easily, without pain or discomfort, something most people take for granted. I start to walk around the bedroom, not the usual slow shuffle but proper walking which increases in speed until I am running around the room shouting excitedly. Anna, who has just been rudely awoken, cannot understand what is going on. I stop and look at her, the penny drops and we both just smile at each other. This, despite me crossing my fingers and rubbing my lucky rabbit's foot, was to be a one-off experience. However, with this event occurring 5 days after an infusion, it must mean something? GDNF or Placebo?

Around the same time the strong solvent/metallic smell returns and fades away again after a few days.

Week 12

I attend the Brain Centre on the 7th of October for an infusion and to complete various questionnaires. The trial team are not interested in my waking up experience, again its qualitative evidence and the trial needs quantitative evidence.

Week 16

Today, the 4th of November, I am at the Brain Centre for an infusion and Medical Illustrations for an off-medication assessment. I complete various questionnaires and have my blood taken.

I report the smell again as an adverse event.

Week 20

At the Brain Centre again, on the 2nd of December, everything starts well, blood pressure under control. But 40 minutes into the infusion Yolanda notices the pump pressures are slowly building and one by one the pumps are shutting down. I have only had 40 minutes worth of infusion.

The team kindly offer me the opportunity to redo the week 20 infusion, I jump at the chance. So, it is arranged for the 8th of December, it has to be within a week to be in line with the trial protocol.

I arrive and meet S, an engineer from Renishaw, the company who manufacture Steven Gill's infusion device and ports. He is here in case the pumps fail again, strangely he is not wearing a boiler suit and there is no sign of oil on his hands.

Yolanda comes up with the idea of reclining the seat so gravity can help with the infusion, it seems to work as this time the infusion is successful. I report the smell again.

Mihaela has been given a Christmas pudding, she does not know what to do with it or when to eat it.

Week 24

8.30 a.m., the 5th of January at Medical Illustrations again for an off-medication assessment. It's not so much of a problem being 'off' any more. I ask Jeanette to check if there is any movement in my right arm swing. She reviews the tapes from today which shows there is a slight movement, but not as much as the left arm. Some is better than none, so that is great. Back to the Brain Centre for another infusion of what must be GDNF. We are still not encouraged to talk with the other participants, it seems a bit rude sitting next to someone and hardly talking. Usually it is the same people every time, obviously, the trial team do not want to mix us up too much.

Week 28

On the 27th of January 2016 I am sitting in the infusion room, midway through my infusion, when Dr Whone, or Alan as it is now, walks in with some medical students trailing in his wake. We greet each other and he asks if he can examine me to demonstrate the procedure to the students, I agree and he begins.

'Hold your arms out in front of you.' He says.

After a minute or so of watching intently he says 'Now bring them to your face.' After a minute or so he looks at me and I say 'I know.'

Then he introduces me to the students saying 'This is Mr Rollin and he used to have a tremor.'

I am delighted, it confirms what I have known for weeks I am definitely on GDNF. My tremor has improved to such an extent that it is hardly noticeable, it is amazing.

Week 32

Another off-medication assessment with Jeanette and Andrew. We walk back to the Brain Centre and pass Lucy, the senior research nurse, I have not seen her for weeks so I say 'Good Morning.'

She replies but looks a bit vague. Later whilst I am having my infusion, she comes into the infusion room and apologises 'You are looking so well; I did not recognise you.'

It's a nice thing to say.

I report the metallic/solvent smell again as an adverse event. I keep telling the team about all the good improvements that I have noticed but there is still the qualitative problem.

Week 36

Another uneventful infusion on the 22nd of March. Yolanda's idea about reclining the chairs still works, if the pressures starts to build, we recline the chair and the pressures reduces over a few minutes.

Week 38

PET scan day, it's the 5th of April 2016. A year since they tried to sort my heart out by performing a chemical cardioversion, well that didn't work. But this GDNF certainly does, I am off-medication for the PET scan and I feel great. Anna is going with me today, so we get ready and travel to the Brain Centre. Sitting in the waiting room is John who I last saw at the test infusion, he has stayed overnight at the Holiday Inn.

He tells us he is a little worried as the bar staff at the hotel did not need to be told what his order was last night.

He's getting to be a regular.

We are joined by Caroline, a nurse who is helping out the trial team as they're so busy.

The taxi arrives and off we go, I am not at all drowsy and listen to the conversation. I am to be first in today, so as we approach the hospital, Caroline gives me some of the required medication.

I am not at all worried about the scan, I will sleep like last time. We arrive and Caroline leads the way. She does not know the short cuts so it is a slightly longer walk than before, but that's OK as I am feeling fine. When we get there, it is a quick kiss for Anna and I am straight in to be prepared. They ask if I want to be sedated which I refuse so I am ushered into the scanner. I ask if perhaps they could put the radio on for me, 'no problem' I am told. At 10.50 a.m. everything is ready and the table slides into the machine, it reminds me of a DVD loading, the radio is on and I'm comfortablish.

The scanner starts and immediately the radio is drowned out, I can just about make out the odd snippet of music. So, I close my eyes to sleep, but I can't, I am wide awake. This bloody GDNF! I have improved so much that, unlike last time, I am not tired. I lay there, have 10 or 15 minutes gone yet? I have no idea, there is nothing to gauge time by. No clock and I cannot hear the radio, just odd bits of clarity amongst a sea of noise.

My legs start to seize up and I can feel a twitch forming in my knees. I try to fight it; I must not move or they will have to start again. I must not move! what is the time? I think, I came in at 10.50 a.m., it's going to take an hour and a half, so I should be finishing at 12.20 p.m.

The radio was tuned to Radio 2. Jeremy Vine starts after the 12.00 news, if only I could hear the radio. I strain my ears to hear against the noise. My legs are beginning to hurt, I am going to move, then suddenly I hear the Radio 2 news music. Great it must be 12.00, I wait to hear Jeremy Vine's voice but when it comes it is a woman's voice. Am I confused, what is the time? I am going to move! How long is it since I heard the news start? I do not know. Suddenly, like the relief of Mafeking*, the table is moving, I can feel hands unstrapping me, it is over. It was the worst sort of bush tucker* trial you could imagine and I nearly say. 'I am a participant, get me out of here.'

I shuffle out of the scanner. The staff must have realised I was in trouble because there, waiting for me is Anna with my medication, I have never been so pleased to see her.

We wait for John to have his scan and then we are homeward bound. It turned out that Sarah Cox was standing in for Jeremy Vine.

Week 39

I am nearing the end of the double-blind trial so the delivery system needs to be checked to confirm that it is still working. So, it's straight to Gate 19 at 8.15 a.m. for an MRI scan. Then back to the Brain Centre for a test infusion, before returning to Gate 19 for another MRI scan.

I am escorted back to Gate 19 by Louise, the trial manager. I have to wait my turn so we chat about the trial in general, things that have happened, things that are going to happen. I tell her about some of my experiences, I start and she is stuck, with no chance of escape until I am called for my scan, but she seems interested in what I am telling her.

The scan finished, we return to the Brain Centre and the scan is checked. It's all fine, no problems, the equipment is still delivering the goods*.

Week 40

The 18th of April, this is it the last week of the first trial. What a whirl wind of adventure it has been, full of highs and lows, mostly highs. I am going into the Brain Centre for a day of assessments.

Yolanda carries out the tests with me these include questionnaires on; impulsive/compulsive behaviour, non-motor symptoms and psychological assessments, quality of life, smell test, memory/thinking tests and finally blood tests. I complete all of the tests without any problems.

I return the following day for the last off-medication assessment of the double-blind trial. This is the half way point and I feel so much better than before the trial, I wonder what the next 40 weeks will bring. Jeanette is waiting for me at Medical Illustrations, we complete the assessment and return to the Brain Centre to have a medical examination with Mihaela. She asks if I would like to continue into the Extension trial.

I say 'Can't wait to start. Guaranteed GDNF, yes please.'

The extension trial

Week E0

On the 26th of April, I start the extension trial and everyone is guaranteed to receive GDNF infusions, no change for me then. I am convinced that I have been receiving it throughout.

There have been so many improvements, particularly with my walking; not only have I sped up, but the shuffling has gone. My Mother has commented that before the trial, she always knew when I was walking down the side entrance to her house as she could hear me shuffling and dragging my feet. Now she cannot differentiate between me and other visitors.

Before the trial, I had to obtain a special mouse for the computer as my tremor made it extremely difficult to manage. I was constantly having to correct mistakes caused by the mouse moving randomly. When typing I would enter the same letter several times and then have to go back to erase the repetitions.

Now I can easily use a standard mouse and repetitions are rare. My hand writing is now larger and more importantly, legible. Over the last few months, I could be sitting quietly or performing some task when suddenly I realise that; my arm has not shaken for a while, that I can smell the coffee that I am drinking, that I can taste my food. If I meet someone who I have not seen for a few months, they generally comment on how much better I look. It cannot all be the Placebo effect.

After my pre-trial off-medication assessment, I thought that I would be forced to give up work within a few years. Now, if I can continue to receive infusions, I am confident that I can work until a normal retirement age.

My first guaranteed GDNF infusion begins, the pumps play up a bit but recover when the chair is reclined. It feels no different to the previous infusions but as a precaution I have to stay 3–4 hours after, just in case I am a GDNF virgin. I report the smell again, it happens 2–3 days after every infusion and gradually fades over a week or so. I do not know if this is common with the other participants as we still are not allowed to talk about the trial.

Week E4

The 24th of May, an uneventful infusion. I reported a new adverse event, that I am getting a pins and needles sensation, all over my body particularly in my neck.

Week E8

On the 28th of June, I have an off-medication assessment at Medical Illustrations followed by an uneventful infusion at the Brain Centre.

It is the 29th of June 2016, and I have received an email from the trial team. They want to organise a telephone conference with the participants to release some brief initial results. It's happening on the 7th of July at 1.00 p.m. We are reminded that all aspects of the trial are confidential. We may be approached by journalists and if so, we are to refer them to the Parkinson's UK press office, as they are coordinating the publicity. They would like some of the participants to share their 'stories' and ask us to contact them if we are interested.

I am more of a sit back and watch sort of person. However, I am so amazed at my improvements that I want to be involved, people should know about this wonder drug. So, I send an email with a few of my highlights. I received a reply the next day from H at Parkinson's UK. She's very interested in my story and we make arrangements to speak after the results are announced.

I take a day off work on the 7th of July to ensure I do not miss the telephone conference; I connect to it just before 1.00 p.m. and I am confronted by a barrage of noise as everyone is speaking at once. S from Parkinson's UK calls everyone to order and the voices subside. He then introduces Alan, who thanks various people for their work on the trial and runs through a brief summary of the workings of the trial.

He then announces that 'the trial did not meet the primary efficacy endpoint.'

What does this mean?

He goes on to explain that; unfortunately, there was not a significant difference in improvement between the placebo and non-placebo groups. Meaning that the trial has failed. However, this is only part of the results and it is going to be months before the full results will be released.

I am devastated. How could this be when I have improved so much. The full results will prove GDNF's worth, they must be better, it cannot just be me, can it?

I email Alan to thank him for the way he delivered the results, I do not hear back from H.

Week E12

It's the 19th of July, back at the Brain Centre for an infusion with symptom and psychological assessments. The mood in the infusion room is low, Yolanda takes my blood pressure only to discover that my heart rate is 130, my irregular heart rhythm is back. Mihaela and Sonali, the other trial doctor, discuss the situation with Alan. It's decided to perform an ECG* on me, by the time this happens my heart rate is reducing so we proceed with the infusion.

95

It's the 26th of July and I have just had a phone call from Sonali, the trial team have been discussing me and they feel that the infusions maybe putting a strain on my heart, they want to suspend them. I am horrified, this is the last thing I want, I argue the fact that I do not have any symptoms and I would prefer to carry on. She says that the trial team will discuss it and get back to me.

Two days later I receive an email from the trial team. They are asking me to attend the Brain Centre the day before my next infusion and early on infusion day for an ECG to ensure I am fit to continue.

I arrive as requested for the first ECG* Yolanda's not in yet. She arrives a few minutes later full of apologies, she carries out the ECG, all fine.

Week E16

The 16th of August, I am at the Brain Centre extra early to have the ECG, which

Jeanette carries out, today my heart is behaving itself, it's fine. We hurry over to Medical Illustration for the off-medication assessment. No problems as expected. There really is no difference between 'on' and 'off' periods any more. Back to the Brain Centre for an infusion followed by memory / thinking assessments and a blood test.

Week E20

On the 15th of September, I have another uneventful infusion. I am still getting the pins and needles as well as the smell.

Week E24

It is the 11th of October. I am going to Medical Illustrations for an off-medication assessment followed by an infusion. Yet again everything goes off without a hitch, as they say 'it's only brain surgery.'

Week E28

On the 8th of November. I have another infusion at the Brain Centre. We have to recline the chair as the pump pressures were increasing. I am still reporting the smell and the pins and needles sensation. My Parkinson's really is just an inconvenience at this point.

It's the 11th of November, Alan sends an update letter to all the participants. The letter informs us that the top-line analysis, which was released in July, was very limited. It only looked at the performance on certain movement tests and did not take into account other data which is still being worked through. Once this is completed there is going to be a meeting with Pfizer and all the other interested parties to agree the next steps. This may include a longer-term extension study for the existing participants. They would also like to hear our input regarding an end of study event.

Week E32

It's the 6th of December. I attend Medical Illustrations for an off-medication assessment followed by infusion, once again it's uneventful which is nice. I would gladly swap this sort of 'Groundhog Day*' with Bill Murray.

On the 20th of December I receive an email to inform me that the event, to mark the end of the trial, is going to be on the afternoon of Sunday the 5th of March at The Bristol Hotel in Prince Street. This is lucky as we are booked to go away on holiday the next day.

I received, on the 23rd of December, an email update from Alan to telling us that following a meeting with Medgenesis and Pfizer in New York, Pfizer's scientific and clinical members are going to recommend to their decision makers to proceed with a further trial.

Week E36

The 6th of January 2016, an infusion at the Brain Centre. I have put weight on over Christmas, Yolanda tells me off and then offers me some chocolates.

Week E39

The 25th of January. I am back at Gate 19 for MRI scan, then over to the Brain Centre for a test infusion, before returning for second MRI. All is fine.

Week E40

It is the 30th of January 2017 at the Brain Centre. I am here for a series of assessments including a hand–eye coordination test on a laptop. Mihaela is concerned that my tremor may affect the results and questions if I am fully 'on' and if I feel OK to carry on. I start the test and Mihaela busies herself with some paperwork, I continue with the test and I am aware that Mihaela has left her paperwork and is watching me intently. I complete the test and she express surprise that I've done so well considering my tremor. I explain that if I want to, I can now stop my tremor.

The 31st of January this is the last day ever of the trial. My last ever off-medication assessment with Jeanette and Andrew, we complete the assessment. I bid Andrew goodbye and thank him for his help over very nearly 2 years. Jeanette and I walk back through the atrium to the Brain Centre, talking about our shared adventures, we say goodbye. Alan carries out a physical examination and an ECG, we chat about the possibility of further trials. It is hopeful that the participants will continue to receive infusions as part of an ongoing safety trial to be run alongside the proposed phase 3 trial. We gather in the corridor and it's goodbye to Alan, Mihaela and Yolanda.

The trial has become such a large part of my life. Over the last 80 weeks the trial team has merged with the participants to become a GDNF coalition, with all of us working together to hopefully prove that GDNF is indeed a wonder drug.

I am going to miss my visits, as I leave the Brain Centre, I am saddened that the trial is over but pleased that I was part of it and convinced that GDNF will move onwards and become a treatment for Parkinson's and maybe other Neurological conditions.

THE GATHERING AND MY RESULTS

I received an email today, the 17th of February, from Alan to tell us that Pfizer remain on track to make their decision by the end of February. Alan also mentioned that if Pfizer do not proceed then Medgenesis will be looking for alternative funding.

Once all the individual data is finalised, Alan will go through with each of us how we, personally did in the trial. We will also be told whether or not we were on GDNF or placebo for the first 9 months.

Unfortunately, by March Pfizer remain undecided.

It's Sunday the 5th of March, Anna and I drive into Bristol and park by the Harbourside to attend the GDNF event at the Bristol Hotel. It is a bright sunny day and we walk from the car park to the hotel.

Greeted by C from Parkinson's UK, she gives us name badges and we wander through into the function room which is nearly full. I look around and apart from trial team members, I recognise about 6 or 7 participants. This is the first time that the participants have been allowed to socialise. I wonder if all that collective GDNF will cause any seismic activity but things remain stable.

It's a nice friendly gathering, with people forming small groups with fellow participants they have shared the infusion room with. Tea and coffee are being served and we talk with one of the media team from Parkinson's UK about my experiences. Alan comes over and ushers us across the room to meet someone, it is a participant called Ros and her husband Andrew.

She had asked Alan to point me out as she is one of my mother's friends, who I have never met before, she has also experienced improvements over the course of the trial. Alan returns and takes me back across the room and introduces me to two gentlemen, the Chairman and Medical Consultant from Medgenesis. Alan relates my improvements to them and they respond by telling us how committed they are to pushing GDNF forward. We chat with Yolanda, Jeanette and Mihaela and are then seated for a light lunch.

After lunch the speeches begin, it's all very informal and pleasant. One of the participants reads a poem she has written about her life with Parkinson's. I find myself nodding in agreement as she describes the practicalities of various daily tasks. Alan talks about the trial in general and the hopes for the future. A lady called Jemima shows us a section of the documentary that she is making about the trial, there are speeches from; S at Parkinson's UK, Steven Gill's wife, the Medgenesis's chairman, Renishaw and from one of the Participants, Tom Issacs, who although clearly 'off' holds the room in his hands with his witty and insightful words.

I was to discover later the major role Tom had played in the GDNF story, and of his work with Steven Gill to make the phase 2 trial a reality. Thank you, Tom.

It was then time for the photos, including; participants, participants with the team, participants and partners and everyone. It has been a wonderful afternoon.

On the 18th of April 2017, it has been decided to release some of the findings from the study as a whole. This will happen at the annual meeting of the

Movement Disorders Society in June, which is taking place in Vancouver. There is also to be another telephone conference, when Alan will be in a position to give more detail from the analyses of both trials.

On the 19th of April I receive a phone call from Hannah, the research administrator, she makes an appointment for me with Alan for the day after tomorrow to discuss my personal results.

I arrive at the Brain Centre for 1.00 p.m. on the Friday. Anna is working but she has made arrangements to come over when I go in. Yolanda and Lucy are there and tell me Alan is running an hour or so late, no surprise. A while later Yolanda comes and tells me that 'Alan is in the building'. I text Anna and she arrives just as I am going in. Alan greets us warmly and as usual apologies for being late. To start with he asks how I am getting on as it has been a while since my last appointment with him.

Then we get to the interesting part, he asks what I thought I was on for the double-blind trial; GDNF or placebo. I respond, 'without a doubt GDNF.' He pauses for a second and then confirms that, yes, I was indeed on the GDNF. I knew it, this confirms that all my improvements are real and not due to the placebo effect. He then proceeds to give me a few of my individual results, which only refer to the off-medication assessments carried out with Jeanette at Medical Illustrations, each part was repeated twice and averaged out in order to improve the accuracy.

Off-medication assessments results week 0 – week E40, 80 weeks in total.

Part 2 UPDRS off-medication 45% improvement

Part 3 UPDRS off-medication 45% improvement

Left finger taps 1ˢᵗ attempt 97% improvement

Left finger taps 2ⁿᵈ attempt 77% improvement

Right finger taps 1ˢᵗ attempt 128% improvement

Right finger taps 2ⁿᵈ attempt 106% improvement

Timed walk 1ˢᵗ attempt 37% improvement

Timed walk 2ⁿᵈ attempt 35% improvement

I quickly average out the results and I am amazed, 71% improvement over the duration of both parts of the trial week 0 – week E40.

I ask Alan 'Has my Parkinson's been reversed?'

To which he replies 'Yes'

Words fail me, Anna and I both look at each other and smile.

Alan then goes on to say that I had been one of the better responders to GDNF. But unfortunately, some participants did not do as well. I am dumbfounded, I knew that I had improved but I did not realise by how much.

We had set out to discover if GDNF could slow, stop or reverse the progression of Parkinson's, in my case it did slow, it did stop and it did reverse my Parkinson's. I wonder out loud what would happen if I could continue to receive infusions. The answer, we don't know.

This has been a day that I shall remember for the rest of my life. I will be boring people with my results for many years to come. Opportunities like this do only occur once in a life time and I am so glad that I had the chance to participate.

Part 2 UPDRS off 45% improvement

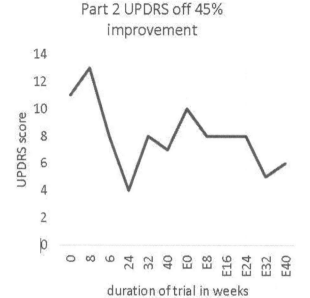

This assessment relates to 'Motor Aspects of Experiences of Daily Living' and includes speech, chewing & swallowing, dressing, hygiene, handwriting, freezing, turning in bed and other tasks. Each section is scored with normal being 0 to severe problems being 4. Out of a total of 100, the higher the score the more difficulties you are experiencing.

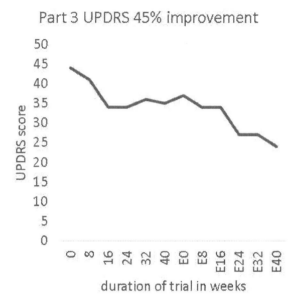

Part 3 UPDRS 45% improvement

Part 3 is scored the same as part 2, but tests 'Motor examinations' including facial expressions, rigidity, gait, hand movements, arising from a chair, postural stability, posture and tremor.

left finger taps 87% improvement

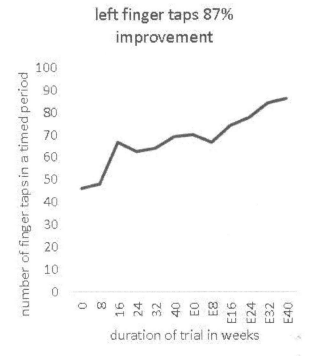

With this assessment you are seated with a small table positioned in front of you. On the table there are 2 marks roughly 40cm apart, using the index finger on either your left or right hand you have to tap the table alternating between the marks moving as quickly as possible, ensuring you actually touch the marks until the allotted time is up. The assessment is carried out twice for each finger with the results averaged.

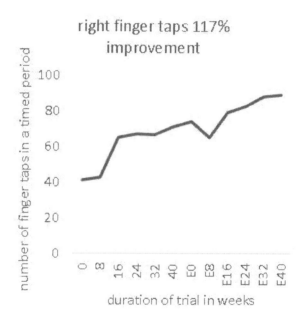

right finger taps 117% improvement

timed walk 36% improvement

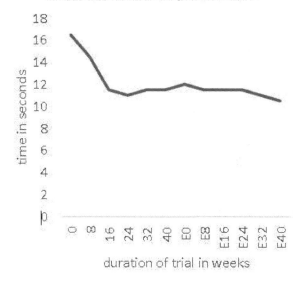

With this assessment you walk as quickly but safely, as you can between positions marked on the assessment room floor while being timed. Again, the assessment is repeated and then averaged. These results confirm the improvement in walking I experienced at week 8 on the Road to Damascus*.

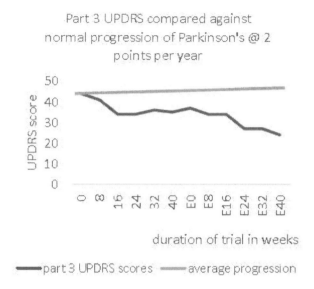

Part 3 UPDRS compared against normal progression of Parkinson's @ 2 points per year

duration of trial in weeks

part 3 UPDRS scores ━━ average progression

This graph clearly illustrates the difference between what my UPDRS score actually was at week E40 and what it would have been expected to be over the time period of the trial. As Parkinson's normal progression is 2 points per year, without the trial my score should be 47, it was actually 24 or you could say my deterioration has been delayed by maybe 10 years.

THE DESCENT

The 25th of May 2017, I receive an email from Alan giving details of the telephone conference, which is being held on the 5th of June at 3.00 p.m. to give us more trial results.

Alan is going to be in Canada. The group data from the trials is to be presented at the International Meeting. We are again warned that this information is confidential and that we must not share it with anyone.

Thinking that the full results are close to being published I contact C at Parkinson's UK to see if they would like to hear my story, she passes my details on the media team.

I come home early so I can join the telephone conference; I connect just before 3.00 p.m., it's the usual chaos before S from Parkinson's UK calls for order and everyone settles down. He starts by giving us the sad news that Tom Issacs had passed away, across the phone line there is a hush as the news sinks in to the participants who knew him. GDNF has lost its knight in shining armour.

The call is passed over to Alan who expresses his condolences, after a moment or two he begins to give us a breakdown of the results. He acknowledges that the results do not reflect how many of the participants felt they had improved, and that the scoring system used could be failing to record some of the improvements. However, he states that it has to be used to ensure that the scientific community accept the results. The results show that GDNF is no better than existing drug treatments. I think, maybe, but existing drug treatments only mask the symptoms where as GDNF is

an attempt at restoring the damage
caused by Parkinson's.

He moves on to highlight the successes of
the trial; crossing the blood brain barrier,
proving that GDNF infusions can be safely
tolerated, proving that the delivery system
works. He closes by telling us of the
promising PET scan results which show an
increase in brain activity.

There is a question session, but the
background chatter is increasing so S
brings the call to an end.

On the 26th of July I am admitted to
Southmead Hospital to have my appendix
removed. This is where I had my delivery
system fitted, during the pre-operative
preparation I am asked about previous
operations. I mention having been on the
trial, but no one has heard of it and they
have to google GDNF to discover what I
am talking about. If the people working in
the same hospital which ran our 'ground

breaking' trial do not know about GDNF, how is the world at large expected to know?

On the 4th of August Alan emails to say that the two papers, one for each trial, are nearly ready to be submitted for publication. Again, we are reminded about confidentiality. Pfizer still have not made any decision about developing GDNF further. Medgenesis are in discussions with them and remain hopeful.

Personally, I'm still feeling well. Not as good as when I was on the trial but better than I would have been if I had not been on it.

On the 24th of August I have an Outpatient Appointment with Alan at 9.15 a.m. I am looking forward to seeing him, hopefully he can give me a positive update. I am seen by his registrar, Harry. A very helpful and reassuringly friendly doctor. He tells me that they are all still working towards further trials with GDNF. I tell him that I continue to feel well and have no major problems. No changes are made to my medication.

It's now December 2017. I have just had an update from Alan. I have started to call emails from Alan a 'Paul Daniels*' as in 'you're going to like it, not a lot.'

This one informs us that the two papers have now been submitted one in August the other in September, publication is now expected next year, 2018. Medgenesis are still chasing Pfizer for a decision, with little success.

I am feeling awful, I have deteriorated rapidly since October, the GDNF has definitely worn off; I've started getting some involuntary movement, I have lost 2 stones in weight over the last 4 months without trying, my tremor has returned, I feel fatigued most of the time, with slower movement overall, more shuffling, stooping and I have had a couple of episodes of 'freezing.' This is a common symptom of Parkinson's, you suddenly feel like your feet are glued to the ground and you cannot move, it can last anywhere from a few seconds to several minutes.

Knowing that there is no chance of an appointment, at short notice with Alan, I contact the local Parkinson's nurse. She arranges an appointment for the 2nd of January at 2.00 p.m. I have to go to Cossham Hospital. We have a long talk about my symptoms and she increases my dose of Carbidopa/Levodopa by an additional 2 tablets.

On the 8th of January 2018 I receive an unexpected email (sorry a Paul Daniels*) from Alan to say that before Christmas Medgenesis were told by Pfizer that they would not be going forward with GDNF. Medgenesis were waiting for written confirmation of this, but today one of the participants found an online statement

issued by Pfizer to confirm that they are
no longer pursing any research into new
treatments for Parkinson's.

This confirms to me what has really been
crystal clear for a long time but we have
been blinded by hope. Pfizer have made
the calculations and there will be a quicker
or better return on their investment if
they spend the money on other projects,
never mind the future for Parkinson's
sufferers.

Apparently, Medgenesis have an ongoing
plan, but things do not sound promising.

It is the 14th of January, someone called
John T has sent me an email. He is one of
the participants. I do not know how he got
my email address but that does not
matter. Six of the participants have got
together following Pfizer's announcement
that they are abandoning all research into
new drugs for Alzheimer's and Parkinson's.
They feel that there must be something

that we, the participants, should or could be doing, after having received very significant improvements as a result of GDNF.

They want to involve as many of the GDNF trial participants as possible. They believe that the worst thing we can do is nothing and we need to be discussing what we, as a group, can be doing to help push GDNF onwards. I agree to be involved and to share my email with the rest of the group. If nothing else we can share any snippets of news we have.

Very quickly there are 27 participants who have given consent for their e-mail addresses to be shared with the rest of the group. John T contacts Alan to inform him that a large section of the participants are now in contact with each other and are offering assistance to somehow move GDNF forwards. Alan replies, thanking the group for their openness and agrees to discuss the group's offer.

I receive an email from Ros, my Mother's friend. She says that the GDNF treatment has given her life back to her, despite the first 12 months being absolute hell. Since hearing of Pfizer's final decision, she has been left feeling somewhat sad and numb. I reply saying that GDNF had given all of us our lives back, and that after a year of no infusions we are all desperate to get some more. That we must be positive. Such a huge amount of money has been spent and so much work completed for it not to continue, that we just have to be patients who have patience and wait.

John T is asking the participants to send him details of any improvements we may have had which were missed during the trial. Alan has expressed an interest in them, this is the qualitative evidence the trial team did not want before.

My inbox is buzzing with all the emails from fellow participants as they realise that it is now OK to talk. Mainly of how we can push GDNF forwards, I think John T has stirred up a hornet's nest. All of the months of pent up frustration is pouring out. After much debating and various ideas being put forward and then pulled apart, the consensus appears to be; hold fire and support Alan until we know what or who we are fighting.

On the 29th of January, I receive an email from Alan confirming our worst nightmare.

Firstly, he apologises for the very long time it has taken to update us on the final outcome of the GDNF trial. The wait, he says, also bears testament to Medgenesis, Parkinson's UK and The Cure Parkinson's Trust belief in GDNF and the many efforts that have been made to keep the trial alive. He reminds us that the double-blind study failed to reach its primary end point, showing no clear difference between placebo and active treatment at 9 months. Also, that Pfizer had decided not to be involved in the future development of

GDNF, and that had been decided even before the decision to pull away from research into neurodegenerative conditions altogether. Pfizer were clearly struggling to commit to continuing the GDNF programme due to the results of the failed phase 2 trial.

Apparently, this had been a very difficult decision for Pfizer to take. They had been given full access to the data which they very extensively reviewed for over a year. Unfortunately, Pfizer deciding not to be involved in the future development of GDNF meant that Medgenesis have lost the funding they would need for a phase 3 trial. Without a successful phase 3 trial, there will be no way of securing GDNF for anyone with Parkinson's.

He carries on, saying that the PET scan results suggest that GDNF has a biological action. He continues, that some positive video assessments and the continuing improvement in some participant's symptoms during the extension trial had been interesting. However, it is highly unusual for a phase 2 trial which had not met its primary outcome, to be able to progress to phase 3 and that Medgenesis are continuing to fight for GDNF.

If it was possible for a phase 3 trial to proceed it would not be expected to start until autumn 2019 at the earliest. As they would still need approval from the relevant regulatory bodies, raise the funding, manufacture new supplies of GDNF and to set up hospital sites in multiple countries.

It had been hoped, despite the negative results, that solutions would be found quickly enough to allow a further extension study involving current participants. However, as it has been approximately 3 years since we received our final GDNF infusion, the benefit of restarting GDNF after such a long interruption is unknown and may carry new risks.

Therefore, as a consequence of all these facts, it has been decided by all of the organisations involved in the trial that, regrettably, at this stage, there is no realistic possibility for providing GDNF to the current participants in a long-term extension study as previously hoped.

I sit looking at the screen stunned, re-reading it several times thinking maybe I was reading it wrong, but no, every time I read it, the same words were on the screen. No phase 3 trial, no more infusions. I am feeling lousy already and this does not help. I think of Alan sat in his office composing the email, rewriting it again and again trying to put a positive spin on it but failing each time. Then I remember that day in July 2016 when he announced that the trial had not met its primary end point. As an experienced researcher he must have known that was

129

it, game over, but still he fought on trying to secure a further trial when to the scientific world it was already over.

It is a sad day but at the very start we were warned that there was no guarantee of further infusions. I think that if there had been no significant improvements for the majority of the participants, then the failure of the trial could be accepted. But it wasn't like that, most of us had some sort of improvement. If you can walk when previously you crawled, if you had a tremor and it disappeared. How can you accept that the wonder drug is not going to be available to help those sufferers who so desperately need it?

Can we make a difference

My inbox is melting. The group, which now numbers 30 participants plus partners, are all outraged. There are all sorts of suggestions and plans, stopping just short of storming the Bastille*. John T replies to Alan's email on behalf of the group, going through it point by point suggesting alternative proposals.

There are several participants in the group who are starting to emerge as being very proactive. This is excellent as we will certainly need them in whatever develops from the mess we are in now.

The growing theme from the group is that the scoring system and the trial protocol were flawed in some way. Perhaps if a more suitable scoring system can be found then the phase 2 trial could be re-run. The group has not yet found a direction to channel its energies and various proposals are put forward only to be dismissed by other members. It is a very frustrating time, but at least we are in contact, talking to each other, building relationships, understanding more of the background to the trial and more importantly we have a voice. I think of all the uncertainty, the lack of information and false promises since the trial ended are to blame for the dissatisfaction felt by the participants. We need to move on.

It is the 8th of February 2018; I have an Outpatients appointment with Alan today. Unfortunately, he is unwell so his registrar, Harry, is going to see me instead.

He asks 'How are you?'

So, I tell him what I had told the Parkinson's nurse in January, that I was deteriorating, but that the additional medication she prescribed was helping. He suggests increasing another one of my medications.

I reply by telling him 'I have previously tried a higher dose which had resulted in sudden onset sleep.'

So, he suggests another medication which would enhance the effect of my existing medication, but unfortunately most people feel unwell with it.

I reply 'I feel bad enough already without feeling unwell as well.'

We decide not to change my medication, but he says to contact them if things get worse.

The group receives an email from Jayne, whose partner Darren is one of the participants. She calls for the group to stand back, take stock and move forward as a team, not individuals. Ultimately, we all want the same thing. This brings the group to its senses.

John T, who has been spokesperson for the group asks for a volunteer to take over this role. His intention had only been to get people talking. He steps aside and makes room for Jayne, who has kindly offered to become the group's spokesperson.

We will always be grateful to John T for his initiative in contacting some individuals and bringing them together as a group. The group will go on to challenge the outdated protocols and systems, ensuring a better experience for future trial participants.

Bob emails the group to suggest that those within easy reach of Bristol meet up. Some of us agree to meet at Southmead Hospital on Friday the 16th of February at 'High Noon' in the atrium by Costa.

Jayne sets to collecting together the qualitative data that Alan has requested from the group and emails everyone detailing an initial plan of action.

It's Friday, Anna and I wander into the atrium just before the allotted time. There's a small group of people hastily reorganising the seating to form a large circle, while the Costa staff look on slightly intimidated. We go over and introduce ourselves and the group do likewise. There is Lesley, Jeff, Raj and Ros, all of whom I know from the trial, and some new faces Bob, Nick, Ken, with their partners and of course Darren and Jayne.

 We all get our refreshments and sit around getting to know each other. Jayne in the meantime is going from person to person collecting all sorts of information. One thing that strikes me that there are nine people here all with Parkinson's and we are all relatively young, why is it still considered to be an older person's disease? I wonder; is there a collective noun for a group of people with Parkinson's, if not I will suggest 'A Shake.'

Meeting up is a great opportunity, not just to formalise the outline of a plan, but to put faces to names and finally talk to each other about our collective experiences. Raj takes a picture to mark the occasion, which he later emails to me.

Jayne arranges another 'meet up' this time in Newcastle, for the northern participants.

The group have produced a list of questions which C at Parkinson's UK hopes to have answered very soon. Carol, one of the participants, is busy working on her proposal for a fairer scoring system. The core team of the group are working extremely hard trying to push forwards. We are all emailed the questions and answers sheet which C has compiled.

Disappointingly, it comprises mainly of information we've already been given.

An update meeting is arranged at Julia's house on the 16th of April.

Parkinson's UK would like to work with the participant group to gather feedback about all aspects of their trial experience. What was good, bad, challenging and frustrating about the experience? How can they do better in the future? They would like our feedback to help develop clear recommendations that can be used to plan all future clinical trials funded by Parkinson's UK.

C asks Alan to allow us a second individual meeting to discuss our personal results, including seeing and accessing data. Alan has confirmed that he is open to requests but advises that he will need to fit these appointments around his clinical workload.

Some of the participants are starting to have problems with their ports getting infected and feel that there is no support available from the trial team, which has now largely disbanded. The group send a letter to Alan asking for the provision of aftercare for participants.

As a result of discussions with the group Parkinson's UK are going to provide a qualitative researcher, who will assist in developing a qualitative research protocol for future trials. We are hopeful that the group will be able to contribute towards any change and make immediate recommendations for current and future trials. As well as working on driving longer term change to ensure that qualitative data has a respected place in the medical scientific world.

Lucy, from the trial team, is also trying to ensure that there will be better follow up for us all, with our port and delivery systems. We will all be offered the opportunity to have our ports removed.

There have been no updates about the paper being accepted into any journals as of yet, although it has been re-written and submitted.

By July 2018, Carol had spent the last 18 months working to explain the unexplainable results. She is close to finding common ground with the Neurologists. The problem is the reluctance for change and the negative attitude towards any kind of reform.

In September, I have an Outpatient's appointment with Alan at the Brain Centre. I tell him of my decline over the last year or so; that my tremor has returned, I feel fatigued most of the time, my movement is slower overall, I am shuffling more, I stoop and I have had a couple of episodes of freezing. He notices that I have also developed some dyskinesia (involuntary movements) since he last saw me and prescribes some additional medication. He suggests that we could try to increase my dopamine agonist but that may lead to other problems. We discuss having either Deep Brain Stimulation (DBS) or Apomorphine pump infusions.

He tells me 'To contact Lucy to arrange an inpatient admission to assess my suitability for either, if you need to.'

I discuss it with Anna and I decide to wait and see what I am like in a couple of months.

Judging by the group emails lately a lot of the participants are going down the DBS route, it seems like the GDNF magic is vanishing for us. Apparently, the trial papers are waiting to be submitted for publication yet again, this is the third time. It is almost like there is an embarrassment because the trial failed. Surely any sort of result, good or bad, should be published so the scientific community can learn from it. Until these papers are published the documentary cannot be shown.

The group are busy collating an information sheet for anyone who is undergoing DBS.

A shocking email is sent by Jayne announcing her intention to disband the GDNF participant group forthwith. She does not say why, but I suspect her decision is due to resistance to change within the research community, which is making our cause seem hopeless.

 Within days Carol emails her finalised report on trial methodology and a revamped UPDRS test. It's an excellent piece of work, which should fill the gaps left by the current system. Alan is going to work on it with her to try and produce an alternative methodology. This can then be tested on previous trials to see how results are affected. I hope that the scientific community will take it on board.

THE RESULTS

It is January 2019, I am feeling a bit better, around November time I noticed a slight improvement, let's hope it lasts.

On the 4th of February I received an email from Alan stating that at long last the trial results, for the double-blind placebo-controlled part, of the GDNF Clinical Trial have been accepted for publication. This will be in the leading scientific journal 'Brain', and due to be published online on the 27th of February 2019.

This is important because once these results are in the public domain they can be scrutinised by the scientific community and hopefully, a path forward for GDNF can be found.

The second part of the trial, has also now been accepted for publication in the

'Journal of Parkinson's Disease 'and is also being published online on the 27th of February.

The publication of the results means that the documentary that has been filmed during the course of the trials can now be shown.

Securing publication has been a challenge, involving rewriting the publication several times. The problem has been getting the journals to accept publications of studies that do not meet their clinical endpoints.

 This is the news we have been waiting two years for. Hopefully, the publications together with the documentary will produce a renewed interest in GDNF which may lead to funding for the phase 3 trial.

I contact C from Parkinson's UK and offer to share my experiences.

She says 'I think it would be great to be able to share some of your story as a blog.'

She continues 'We could then share it with the Parkinson's community via social media and hopefully it will help to encourage more people to support and take part in research.'

I sit down and remember some of things I had experienced. I put them together entitling it 'My GDNF Moments.' I send it to her. She tweaks a couple of things and emails me to say its ready, so I google 'GDNF, Andy' which takes me to Parkinson's UK website. There it is, my story just waiting to be read at long last. I am so pleased.

The first part of the documentary is to be shown on the 28th of February, the day after the results are published, with the second part to be shown on the 7th of March. Although I am not in it, I am looking forward to seeing it. How did the featured participants fair? Did they have a similar experience to me?

It's the 27th of February, publication day. I receive a large envelope in the post, it is from the trial team and contains a copy of both trials results. At long last they are in my hands. It makes for heavy reading with lots of specialist terminology, but it acts as confirmation that it is alright to speak about the trial.

The trial results are featured in most of the newspapers, so I buy copies to keep. There is a big article in the Radio Times so I buy that as well. It is also on TV; I see Steven Gill and Raj both being interviewed. It is wonderful. There seems to be a genuine interest in our story, which is great. A few weeks ago, I thought it was a story no one would ever hear.

THE DOCUMENTARY

We have invited the family around to watch 'The Parkinson's Drug Trial - A Mircle Cure?'documentary, so I rearrange the furniture, finding extra chairs to use. We end up with the lounge resembling an extremely small theatre, so I put signs on the sofas; stalls, dress circle, upper circle and so on. The chairs at the edge of the room have a restricted view so they have a sign saying so. We have a torch so we can show people to their seats and at the interval Anna is going to come around with the ice creams, we are ready.

As the family arrive, the volume of the conversation steadily builds. I have the TV on in the background and as the documentary starts, I call the family to order. The room becomes silent and everyone watches intently. A few turn away during the operation part and there are a few hushed questions. As it finishes, I receive a text from a friend.

'Wonderful.' It simply says.

Then the questions start. Although the family had experienced the trial second hand through me, none of them had realised the true level of commitment that the involvement had required. We agree to repeat the evening the following week for part 2, but this time with popcorn as well as ice cream.

It's the 7th of March. Today, part 2 of the documentary is being shown. I hope it lives up to the same quality of storytelling as part 1, which was outstanding.

The family gather again, everyone is looking forward to it, even though they already know the outcome. The programme starts and again, like last week, there is silence.

On screen, Alan is delivering the devastating news that the trial failed to meet its primary end point. The sullen and miserable mood of Alan's listeners is reflected in the off-screen room.

The program finishes and instead of last weeks excited questions there is a stillness in the room, which slowly dissolves as the family absorb the painful facts.

Watching the documentaries has been a powerful and emotional experience with the story being told accurately and truthfully.

A few days later I'm browsing the Parkinson's UK website for any further news or articles, I casually look on the forum only to find a series of shall we say, negative reviews of the documentaries;

"I find it appalling that they may have given hope to thousands of people. They should have said from the start that it had failed."

"Whoever made the programme and whoever gave the go ahead to air it should be ashamed of themselves."

"That garbage will have destroyed the hopes of thousands of people."

"...surely Parkinson's UK must have known the outcome of the trial...if so, why didn't they try to stop the programme rather than let us all be given hope???"

"I was appalled by the way that they aired the programme, giving false hope and treating it like a thriller when it impacts so many people with Parkinson's and their families. I have complained to the BBC."

The Parkinson's UK moderation team replied;

"We wanted to ensure that any portrayal of Parkinson's and the GDNF trial was accurate, balanced and fair. We considered the questions and concerns

*that the documentary might raise
throughout the process of providing
support and advice during the filming
process. For example, as soon as we
became aware of the title of the
documentary, we strongly voiced our
concerns that it may raise false hope for
people affected by Parkinson's.*

*Ultimately how the documentary film
footage was edited and presented, and the
title chosen, was a decision made by the
BBC.''*

Parkinson's UK, who throughout the
documentaries have been portrayed as
one of the good guys, now at the first sign
of any criticism, instead of supporting the
documentary makers, they have
withdrawn their head, like a tortoise, back
into their shell.

I am appalled firstly I cannot believe that
anyone living with Parkinson's in one way
or another could fail to see the progress

that had been achieved during the trial and the possibilities that this progress had opened up. I thought that there would be more important things for them to worry about. So, I reply;

"I was one of the participants in the GDNF trial and feel I must defend the documentary, what you saw was exactly what happened all the ups and downs, celebration and disappointment. We may not like the end results but remember this is research, we do something, we learn from it and we move onwards towards the cure.

The results are not the failure you think it is. We know the delivery system works, we know that infusions of GDNF are safe, we have exciting PET scan results. We are several steps closer to a cure. I personally think that GDNF is the way forward, just look around at all the participants who have come forward to tell of their experiences and improvements.

When carrying out research you hope for the best but must except some knock backs, we are learning as we go and the documentary showed this. We would all like the fairy tale ending but this is reality and sometimes reality is disappointing or upsetting.

The documentary accurately showed what actually happened, the upbeat feeling in the trial was shattered by the results and when Pfizer pulled out people were devastated, all the documentary did was show it as it was.

The purpose of the documentary was to raise awareness of Parkinson's and the trial which I think you will agree it did. By showing the 'warts and all' version, the viewing public had a taste of some of the emotions we all experienced. When we started, we did not know how things would develop and the documentary title did have a question mark at the end."

153

I wonder what hope there is for research if people can be so short sighted.

It is March, I heard today that Carol had passed away peacefully on the 19th of February 2019. She had worked tirelessly on challenging the UPDRS that had been used to measure the GDNF trial and was convinced that it was one of the causes of the trial not meeting its primary target.

The world is a sadder place without her.

Lazarus

Starting around November the previous year, my decline had stopped and I began to improve, slowly at first and then building. By January 2019 I have improved so much that Anna and I start Ballroom and Latin dance classes. We go up to three nights a week, which is something I could not have even considered the previous year. Something is happening, but what?

On the 14th of March, Jayne sends me an email, it is so good to hear from her again. She seems to be rejuvenated and has taken on an even bigger challenge than before. Following the screening of the Parkinson's drug trial documentary, Jayne and Darren have started fundraising through 'Funding Neuro' a charity to help fund further investigation into GDNF, Darren has pledged to raise £1,000,000 to kick start a phase 3 trial and Funding Neuro have agreed to ring fence all fundraising specifically for GDNF. As part of this they are organising a summer fundraising event in July. It is going to be a fete/garden party with a live band. What a fantastic idea, they really are special people.

On Monday the 1st of April at 6.00 p.m. Parkinson's UK are going to hold a telephone conference. The purpose of which is to give the participants of the GDNF trial the chance to find out what Parkinson's UK has been doing to support a potential phase 3 study.

On the 22nd of March, an email from Alan arrives to answer the various questions that have been raised. He tells us that Steven Gill continues to fight for GDNF and is putting together a proposal to run a small-scale lead in trial. The hope is that if it is a success, investment will then be available to hold a full phase 3 trial.

Parkinson's UK have asked for questions from the participants for the telephone conference. So, I ask if they want the qualitative information that Jayne collected from the participants, and if there was a possibility of further assessments as I am feeling so good. I think it is the GDNF still working.

I join the telephone conference call with Parkinson's UK, I am profoundly disappointed with the morass of gibberish they present. Jayne manages to squeeze my question in, but I am disappointed with the response that basically I am no longer clinically interesting. The overall impression I get is that apart from an advisory role we are finished with. We are no longer of any use and have been cast aside. It is a harsh reality to hear this.

I decide to email Parkinson's UK to push further about having assessments to investigate further what is happening to me. My first emails are ignored and then I get a reply simply giving me the brush off. So, I try again and get a reply from A who suggests a telephone conference call including his assistant L. We have the call; my main point is that I am experiencing improvements which I cannot explain. I want to know if they can arrange assessments to investigate further as I feel that I may be holding valuable information about GDNF's longevity. The shortened answer is no, there was no provision for it in the trial protocol.

If I had paid a huge amount of money to part fund a trial, I would want to squeeze every possible piece of information that I could out of it. Who knows which piece of information holds the key that may unlock the secrets of Parkinson's? In my mind I liken it to the final scene in the first Indiana Jones* film where a packing case containing 'The Ark of the Covenant' is being placed in a warehouse, the camera pans out to show thousands and thousands of similar packing cases containing who knows what.

At the end of April Anna and I go away for a few days, I have been feeling great with increases in energy and stamina. On the second evening I take my usual dose of Carbidopa/Levodopa at 6.00 p.m., we go to the restaurant. After about 30 minutes I can feel myself swaying and twitching. The waitress comes to take our order and tries to ignore the fact that I appear to be having some sort of fit whilst ordering the soup followed by a medium steak. This is dyskinesia or involuntary movements and it has slowly been getting worse since the new year. However, conversely, I am feeling better most of the time. This sets the tone for the rest of the break and after we return home gradually the involuntary movements start to occur 2–3 times most days. In between I am feeling great.

My next appointment with Alan is in May. When I go, we discuss how I am feeling, which is great apart from the dyskinesia which Alan describes as problematic. He suggests increasing one of my medications, but I am reluctant, as I feel that I take enough drugs already, but he increases my prescription just in case I need it.

By June the involuntary movement has become a regular occurrence, however I have also noticed that it seems to start 30–40 minutes after taking my medication. One particularly bad Friday I come home from work at lunch time feeling awful and decide not to take the rest of the day's doses of Carbidopa/Levodopa. Within a couple of hours all the involuntary movement has stopped completely. I decide not to take any of the medication all weekend, by Sunday evening I have not had any involuntary movement at all. Involuntary movement is one of the listed side effects of Carbidopa/Levodopa.

Over the next few weeks, I fine tune my dosage of Carbidopa/Levodopa 25mg / 100mg, reducing it from 8 tablets a day to 3 tablets a day and increasing the time between them. I very rarely get involuntary movements now, but I remain feeling great with good levels of energy and stamina.

Why is this happening?

The truthful answer is I do not know. However, I believe that the brain cells that grew during the trial have taken the last three years to fully develop, building neurological pathways or whatever. Now they are fully working and producing dopamine. This together with the artificial dopamine that is in my medication results in me 'overdosing' on dopamine. Which I think may be causing the side effect of involuntary movements.

I have no proof of this theory, but to me the qualitative evidence is overwhelming, unfortunately it is not quantitative.

I contact Alan and his registrar rings me back, I tell her what I have done.

I ask 'Is it OK to reduce my medication like this?'

She replies 'That any reduction has got to be a good thing.'

I feel like I have truly risen from the dead.

THE SUMMER EVENT

Jayne and Darren are holding an update meeting at their house, she gives me directions Anna and I set off. We turn off the main road and continue along a leafy lane, past a pub, and turn in to a driveway when the sat nav tells me to, we cross over a bridge and we are there. It is a lovely riverside setting with a large grassed area, it is going to be perfect for the summer event that they are planning.

Darren and Jayne greet us warmly and make us welcome. Some of the other participants are already here, sitting in the shade to protect them from what is turning out to be a glorious, hot, sunny day. We are introduced to Sharon from the charity Funding Neuro, who tells us of the various plans she has to promote Darren's fund raising. Another idea is to have localised press campaigns, where participants can tell their stories and promote fund raising for the long hoped for phase 3 trial.

 Jayne tells the others about my lack of response from Parkinson's UK regarding on going assessments, and of what is becoming the saga of the lead in phase 3 trial. The main topic is of course the upcoming summer event. We have a lovely afternoon.

It is Saturday the 13th of July, the day of Jayne and Darren's summer event. Jayne has been worried about the weather but the day starts cool with a clear sky. Over the course of the morning the sun comes out and by 2.00 p.m. it is lovely. We are going as a group; Anna and I, Chris and his wife Amy, Sophie and her partner and my Mother. We arrive promptly and discover that there are several participants and their partners already here. Darren is dispensing drinks, while Jayne gives final instructions to the small army of their family and friends who have either volunteered or been persuaded to help out. Everyone has a smile on their face.

We guess how many balloons there are in a car, win a prize on the tombola, have a hot dog and sit and watch the world go by. The gardens go right down to the river and there is a constant procession of boats passing by, the crews must be wondering what is going on. The place is filling up and we spend most of the afternoon catching up with each other. Alan and Lucy arrive and are swamped. The documentary is being shown, you can help yourself to the buffet which is plentiful and tasty.

The auction is a success with bids often reaching hundreds of pounds, everyone is having a great time. Jayne takes the microphone to say some words of thanks and introduces Lucy and Lesley, who both speak, the audience is silenced by the passion in their words. The microphone returns to Jayne and she reminds everyone why we are here, running through a brief history of events.

She calls the participants up and I am humbled by her words, Alan gives an impromptu speech, thanking Jayne and Darren not just for today, but for previous events they have hosted to raise money. The band start up and Anna and I jive the night away, pausing only to listen to Darren serenading Jayne.

Our youngsters call it a day around 10.00 p.m. That's the trouble with the youth of today, no staying power. They are exhausted and retire for the night leaving the old folks to fly the flag. It is nearly midnight when the band finish and the day draws to an end. It has been a great success; we have had a wonderful time.

A couple of days later Jayne announces the total raised, which is in excess of £18,000.

FALSE HOPE

It's the 20th of July, Jayne has been in touch. Parkinson's UK would like some of the participants to take part in the first round of Patient and Public Involvement (PPI) feedback on a study protocol for the proposed clinical trial for GDNF. She has kindly asked if I would be interested. The feedback will be collated by L.

Alan and his team have been preparing a protocol, and they now have a draft ready. The protocol has been shaped based on the participants feedback, so it was not wasted after all. They need the protocol to be reviewed by some of us and other PPI volunteers. The feedback they are looking for is on the top line design of the study. Predominantly; the number of participants to be recruited, the length of the study, the number and format of study visits and the outcome measures to be used.

As the protocol develops, they will ask for our input on things such as; consent processes, information flow throughout the trial; particularly at the end, practical aspects of study visits, the surgery and how to improve the experience for all future participants.

They have been listening.

They are working to tight deadlines and need the feedback returned by Monday the 5th of August.

This is a major step; it brings the possibility of a trial forwards. So, I devote the weekend to completing it.

The protocol makes for interesting reading and I notice that they have included a number of the improvements that the group pointed out. I thoroughly enjoy the process; I imagine that I am one of the new participants and think about the various situations that might develop. I then use my trial experience to suggest changes where I think they are necessary. I work all weekend and email it back on the Monday, a week early. I wonder if they will think that I have not put any thought into it.

I receive an email back from L thanking me for such thorough and considered feedback. As additional sections of the protocol become available for review, she will be sure to let me know.

It is August, it appears that the date for the new trial has now slipped to spring 2020. It has been suggested that once the lead in trial is successfully completed and the phase 3 trial is up and running, the phase 2 participants may be able to receive GDNF on Compassionate Grounds. Apparently the 'Early Access to Medicines Scheme' allows patients with life threatening or seriously debilitating conditions to access medicines that do not yet have a marketing authorisation, when there is a clear unmet medical need.

It is likely that funding will be required, but it is something to aim for.

Darren and Jayne now have a website which they are hoping will raise the profile of the GDNF Participant group. This provides a central place to access information and news regarding the cause. It will also act as a portal for donating to Darren's fund raising, Jayne is asking for contributions, so I am going to send her my GDNF story for inclusion.

The website has now been updated. It tells the GDNF story in an easy to understand way and, despite the official results, there is a very positive feel to it. The other participants stories clearly show the range of improvements that many of us have, with so many parallels to my story. The inclusion of the carer's stories is a master stroke, highlighting the support that we, the participants, received and the hell the carers went through. The website will, I am sure, prove to be a huge resource, which all future participants should be made aware of during the consultation process.

Jayne puts me onto a book called 'Monkeys in the Middle'. It is about the previous GDNF trials, I start to read it and I am hooked. I cannot put it down; it answers so many questions that have been running around my head for months. I think maybe it should be made mandatory reading for the new trial participants.

It is now October 2019 and things have gone very quiet on the GDNF front, although we have been reassured that it is still progressing. There have not been any updates or news of any kind. It seems that like the Mayfly, phase 3 has had its day in the sun.

Personally, I continue to improve. Not only am I still happily managing on reduced medication without loss of stamina or energy, I am now sleeping better. Previously I was woken up by the nagging pain in my back after 3–4 hours sleep. I am now sleeping anywhere between 5–7 hours every night, sometimes oversleeping. Although I wake with back pain, I am no longer woken up by the pain, which is a big difference. Unfortunately, I still have not been able to find anyone who is in the slightest bit interested.

If this information is not recorded soon it may be gone for ever. Someone must want to know?

It has been announced that the documentary 'The Parkinson's Drug Trial: A Miracle Cure?' has won the highly regarded Grierson Award for Best Science Documentary.

The judges said 'The winning film stood out for its lean storytelling of a complex subject, its scale and its heart. The film managed to straddle both the science involved with clarity and the emotional, human dimension with real compassion.'

Documentary maker Jemima Harrison paid tribute to Tom Issacs by saying 'We owe so much to Tom Isaacs, both for being the one who invited us to film the GDNF trial in the first place and for being so utterly unflinching in demanding that we document his Parkinson's with such brutal honesty. It was phenomenally brave of him and all the other trial volunteers who put their lives on the line for science. I hope the series has played a role in raising awareness of how very badly a cure is needed and that it will remain a part of Tom's enduring legacy.'

Sentiments that I think we all agree with.

The conference and shine

Parkinson's UK are hosting The Research Support Network Conference 2019 in Solihull on Saturday the 23rd of November. It is basically an update on research that they are involved in and their plans for the future. Jayne and 2 participants, Sharon and Christine, have been invited to give speeches to close the event.

Vicki, another participant, has had a wonderful idea for raising the profile of Parkinson's and the GDNF trial. She has come up with a song, called 'Shine' which has been written and performed for us, with the ultimate goal of securing a Christmas number one hit. It may be a challenge as it is already well into November. Hopefully the song will at least be on the radio and or YouTube, which will be a massive boost to the public's awareness of the trial and Parkinson's in general.

She wants to record the song with as many participants as possible joining in. I click on the link and I am taken to YouTube and the song plays. I listen carefully, it is a catchy song and I like it. Later on, I find myself humming it. This could be a success and will shout a powerful message to the entire Parkinson's scientific community; 'we are aware that you want to forget all about us, but we are still here and we are not going away.'

I email Jayne to wish her well for the conference she casually asks 'How are you?'

I tell of my improvements and how well I am doing.

She replies 'Christ Andy that is absolutely amazing!!'

I am so pleased, someone is interested. It's just a pity she doesn't work for Parkinson's UK.

It is the day of the conference, I am not going, but will watch the video link. I login just as it is starting. I know that Jayne and the others are not on until mid-afternoon, so I settle down to watch the other speakers.

The event is being hosted by A, who I spoke to unsuccessfully about ongoing assessments earlier in the year. There is a link where you can post questions to be answered by some of the delegates later in the day. So, I post a couple of questions about GDNF, I am the first person to post any questions, I notice later that Jayne and Lesley have both posted questions as well.

The speakers are very good but unfortunately all the research that is mentioned is 5–10 years away from clinical use. The questions to be asked list is growing but somehow our questions never move from the bottom of the list. Elvis with his suspicious mind may suspect foul play*. So, when the questions are asked, and ours are completely ignored, I am very frustrated.

Eventually it is time for the speeches. Sharon goes first, followed by Jayne and then Christine. Jayne has been given a 5 minute time slot and her subject is 'Clinical Trials from a Carer's Prospective.' She begins with a brief description of how Darren became involved with the trial, stepping up a gear to talk about the lack of support for the participants once the trial had finished. She squeezes in a mention of Darren's quest to 'Raise a £1,000,000 for GDNF'. Moving on to speak of how disappointed she is that all the speakers today consider that a treatment for Parkinson's is still 5–10 years away and that GDNF has not been mentioned when we, the group, all know it works.

She announces to the audience 'GDNF works, we know it, it is just that science has not proven it yet.'

She calls upon the researchers present to work harder because some people do not have the luxury of waiting another 5–10 years. She has spoken for 15 minutes, easily the most passionate and captivating speaker of the day. She will not be asked to speak again next year and A probably feels like he has gone 10 rounds with Hulk Hogan*.

The conference is quickly brought to a close, the camera is just panning out as an audience member is getting to his feet. He storms the stage grabbing the microphone and demands that the panel come back and answer the posted GDNF questions. The camera link is cut and the screen turns dark.

Jayne's speech has been so provoking that emotions are running high, but it is an emotional subject. It seems that GDNF is a bit like Marmite, only instead of love or hate it we have either believe in it or not believe in it, there is no middle ground. Well done Jayne.

It is Sunday the 24th of November and Vicki emails the group; things are progressing really well with her song and she is trying to organise as many participants as possible to meet up to 'lay down some tracks'. The hospital is the obvious choice of location given all the connections to the group and the trial.

A phone call is made only to be told; filming is not allowed within the hospital grounds.

'What about if it is for charity.' Is the reply.

'Only if it is the hospital charity.' Is the answer.

Once again Darren and Jayne step forward to save the day and arrangements are quickly made. As many participants as possible are required to be at Darren and Jayne's house on the following Wednesday to record the backing for the song and do some filming. Oh, and by the way it is a Christmas theme. It is just like being in 'The A-Team*,' and I love it when a plan comes together.

I arrange a day off work as I feel that any possibility of promoting GDNF and Darren's quest has to be supported. Plus, it is another chance to socialise with the group.

Mid-morning on Wednesday and I am on location, at Jayne and Darren's. I am wearing my Christmas shirt, waistcoat and a Christmas hat. They have decorated the entire house ready for Christmas weeks early, it is very festive and jolly and there is a massive decorated tree in one corner.

There are lots of participants here today all wearing Christmas jumpers and hats.

I am introduced to Vicki, who I once shared an infusion room with, her vision and spirit are why we have assembled here today. With her is Rick, the talent behind the song, who has travelled from Scotland for today. We begin, as usual with a cup of tea, and we go around the room introducing ourselves, this tends to happen at every get together. There is always someone who has not met someone else and it is usually name, rank and serial number. When it is my turn, I give my name, trial number and tell everyone of my continued improvement. Jayne adds that if she refers to participants who are still improving then she means me. A few of the others say that they are still benefiting from GDNF, it is nice to know I am not alone.

The recording session starts with Rick outlining what he would like to achieve, he is anticipating our talent and looks doubtful. The song is played through a couple of times and then we have a practice, Rick is accompanying us with his guitar and is playing it nice and loud, just in case. The smile returns to his face, we are not as bad as he first thought.

We are singing the technical bit so he plays the backing track and when it is our time he nods and the group as a whole sing out; 'wow a wow a wow a wow a wow aaaa AA!!'

Rick's impressed, I do not think he has ever seen so much talent in one room at the same time.

He declares 'You are naturals.'

We sing it through a few more times, he is pleased, so we move onto the filming. One by one we stand in front of Jayne's Christmas tree holding hand written signs. Each sign has only 1 or 2 words on it, each word a facet of Parkinson's. Mine says 'Exhausting.' Very apt, I think.

Then the whole group are filmed standing in front of the tree again. This time we are going to be singing with some of us holding signs, which collectively spell out the message. 'G.D.N.F,' 'Help us to,' 'Bring it back,' 'It works.'

Rick is delighted with the results and we have been quicker than expected. There is an excitement in the room as the group prepare to leave.

Someone asks. 'What shall we call ourselves?' across the room comes the answer 'The GDNFer's.'

The name sticks and that is who we now are. It had been a really good positive day with a surprisingly good turnout of participants. It just shows how important the cause is to all of us, it reminds me of the feeling of achievement I had during the trial. The one good thing that has come out of our abandonment is the way a group of strangers who believe in something so passionately they have joined forces to devote time and energy attempting to give their story the fairy tale ending it deserves.

Vicki and Rick spend the next few days and nights working away editing our filming, combining it with other footage sent in from around the world, blending our singing efforts to produce 'Shine' by 'The GDNFer's'. Unfortunately, it was not the Christmas number one that Vicki had hoped for, but who can compete with a song about a sausage roll.

The process had revived the group and given us our anthem, which I was especially pleased about as my suggestion would have been 'Don't give up on us' by David Soul*. The chorus 'Stand up' 'Shout out' 'Be counted' became our tag line and it did add just under £3,000 to Darren's total.

The day reminded us of how important it is for the group not just to plot our next move but to socialise with each other, the idea of a reunion was born.

The end game

The 4th of December 2019, I have an Outpatient's appointment with Alan. Anna and I wait the usual hour or so, then he calls us in. I am feeling on top of the world and tell him so. He is pleased that I have improved, I mention my theory, he listens but does not comment. Alan then explains to me that when the nerve endings die off in Parkinson's the result is more dopamine going through the remaining nerve endings. He likens it to a football crowd passing through two turnstiles; if you close one turnstile, then more people have to pass through the remaining one. This can mean stronger doses of dopamine which could explain my 'overdosing' effect.

I say to him 'I understand that, but it does not explain my increased stamina and energy, or my improved walking or my improved tremor or my improved sleeping and general wellbeing.'

'No' He replies.

I feel so good I think that I could give Steve Austin* a run for his money.

Communications from Parkinson's UK have been strained since the conference; there are questions that remain unanswered, promises that have not been kept, concern over their duty of care to participants, lack of any sort of support structure, physical and mental, for the participants and the lack of promised support to continue our quest to improve the participant experience.

Do Parkinson's UK think it is reasonable to leave trial participants with a head full of highly technical equipment with no provision for its removal or after care?

Jayne writes a strongly worded letter to Parkinson's UK on behalf of the group, 20 of the participants sign it, in the hope that 3 years after the trial finished Parkinson's UK will face up to its responsibilities.

Jayne receives confirmation of receipt together with a promise to respond within 5 days.

The reply, when it arrives it is full of generalisations and 'passing the buck.'

They are concerned to hear that we feel let down by the charity, but the trial team at Southmead Hospital are responsible for providing ongoing medical support and care to participants. They also understand, from Southmead Hospital, that all participants have been advised by the study team that it is their choice whether to have the ports and delivery device removed or not.

They say that they do encourage people developing new trial proposals to consult with the participants group from the previous GDNF trial when developing their proposals.

Parkinson's UK agree that it may have been valuable to continue to assess participants to help understand the longer-term effects of GDNF. Unfortunately, this was not included in the original protocol and therefore cannot be added.

Parkinson's UK add that they would welcome the opportunity to meet with us to discuss these points in more detail.

Our first reunion is going to take place at the end of January/first weekend in February at the Holiday Inn in Filton. This venue has been chosen due to many of the participants staying there during the trial. Parkinson's UK have been offered the opportunity to attend the Saturday session of the reunion so we can talk face to face.

Friday 31st January 2020, it is the reunion. We only live a few miles from the Hotel but are staying over in order to be able to socialise more. Anna and I arrive at 2.30 p.m. and check in, we go to our room, and drop our bag off and return downstairs and wander over to the bar area.

The first thing we see is Jayne collecting chairs and tables as they are vacated in order to form 'The Parkinson's Circle', which at this stage, takes up a third of the floor area with the potential to grow even bigger. We go over and greet my fellow participants and their partners who have, by now, become friends. We catch up and ask after each other, this is to be the social side of things, we spend a pleasant afternoon happy in each other's company. By now the circle has become an untidy oval. Darren has a word with the bar staff and they find a room into which we disappear, leaving the bar staff to restore the bar to nicely ordered squares.

We take the opportunity to begin planning for the business side of things, our

meeting with Parkinson's UK. We need
some answers to our grievances, to
restore our relationship with them and to
get a commitment for the long hoped for
phase 3 trial. Jayne goes around the room
asking what every participant would like as
an outcome from Saturday. It is the same
as it has always been; support, resources,
ongoing assessments, a more accurate
scoring system for trials, a phase 3 trial,
openness and honestly. All of which have
been promised but for various reasons
never delivered.

We settle down and are formulating an
agenda when we are given shock news,
the long hoped for phase 3 lead in trial is
likely to be delayed yet again, apparently
the companies involved cannot agree
terms. If this trial does not start soon then
it may never start, what is wrong with
these people. They have all invested time,
money and expertise, if this trial fails to
even happen then not only do people with

Parkinson's suffer but there will be little chance of any return on their investment. It is asked what we as a group can do to push things along; ask Parkinson's UK if they will review the protocol early is the answer, as this will knock a few months off the required time and give some breathing space.

This will have to be added to the agenda.

The day has triggered all sorts of memories for me, some good, some bad. It has been a long journey and we are I hope nearly at our destination. If we were travelling from Bristol to the North Pole, I think we have reached The Arctic Circle with Anna as my Eskimo guide. We battle against the cold and keep a watch for Polar Bears, but at least we are 'Inuit' together.

Saturday morning, we get up early and have breakfast, Anna is working so I drop her off and return to the hotel. The meeting starts at 10.00 a.m., the group has an hour and then we are joined by Parkinson's UK. We have the usual introductions and when it is my turn, I give my name and trial number.

Then tell them that 'I am the pain in the arse who believes that I am still improving.'

 The meeting begins with Jayne asking if they can give us an update on the current position regarding the lead in trial.....

And that is where my account ends. Perhaps not where you either expected or wanted it to end, but where it has got to end. As you have probably realised there are not many happy ever after endings in the clinical trial world.

If you think that this ending is a bit abrupt or maybe even frustrating, I agree. Welcome to 'Never, Never Land.'

193

Déjà vu

Déjà vu - a feeling of having already experienced the present situation.

In 2004, a company called Amgen terminated their clinical trial of GDNF for Parkinson's.

This Phase II trial did not meet its principle endpoints at 6 months, it was a 'failure.' GDNF had been considered to be one of the most promising treatments in development for Parkinson's and most of this trial's participants were beginning to experience improvements. A group was formed comprising of trial participants, trial doctors and researchers to persuade Amgen to reinstate treatments for the participants. The statistical analysis had been flawed; there had been a small number of participants, making the trial underpowered and incapable of ruling out the effect of GDNF on Parkinson's disease. The GDNF did not fail, but the trial design and delivery methods did. The group were ultimately unsuccessful in their efforts.

Amgen were later to grant Medgenesis an exclusive, worldwide license for GDNF.

And this is where I began....

AFTER

In my opinion, and it is only my opinion, GDNF has failed to progress as a treatment. Not because the various trials have failed, as there is compelling evidence that it does work, but for various complex business reasons.

At the time of writing this, during the Covid-19 Lockdown in April 2020, GDNF's future remains unclear.

As they say 'When one door closes, another one slams in your face'. Steven Gill, who has been GDNF's champion throughout is exploring different avenues and remains positive. His delivery system, which was proven during the trial, has now been used in the treatment of brain cancer in children, this fact alone makes it all worthwhile.

On a personal level, it is now 5 years since I started on the trial and 3 years 3 months since my last infusion and I remain improved.

I believe the reason this has happened is that the brain cells grown during the trial are now fully functioning. No one seems to have an alternative answer which explains my improvements and the reduction in medication that has occurred. Remember Parkinson's is a degenerative disease.

My symptoms have changed over the years but I am still taking less Parkinson's medication, 7 tablets a day instead of 12 a day. That is 1,825 tablets less per year. I have no idea how long my improvements will last or if there are more to come, but I am extremely grateful for the extra time GDNF has given me.

Why me?

I do not know. Perhaps it is possible that some Parkinson's sufferers respond better to GDNF than others, after all our symptoms can vary. This is one of Parkinson's secrets that we need to understand, but without additional post trial assessments it will remain a secret.

I feel both honoured and proud to have been part of what should have been one of the most important ever medical advances. And saddened that its fate has become a business decision instead of a healthcare one.

After all the highs and the lows, the peaks and the troughs, the joy and the devastation. Would I go through it all again?

Yes, without a moment's hesitation.

Does GDNF work? I know it does, 100%

What do you think?

To borrow some of Jayne's words;

'GDNF works, we know it, it is just that science has not proven it yet.'

To be continued ?.....

Darren and Jayne have a website;

www.raise-a-million-for-gdnf.org

Please visit for more information about Darren's quest, participants stories, news and much more. If my account has made you feel shock, horror, outrage or any other emotion, then you can make a donation through the website, please dig deep.

Vicki's song 'Shine' by The G.D.N.F.er's is available from www.amazon.co.uk

Glossary

Baby Bio - is a concentrated plant feed. Page 17.

BAWA — a Health & Leisure Club on Southmead Road, Bristol. Page 23 &75.

Bob Geldof did not like Mondays — reference to 1979 song 'I Don't Like Mondays' by The Boomtown Rats. Page 55.

David Soul — Starsky and Hutch actor turned singer who had a 1976 hit entitled 'Don't give up on us.' Page 184.

Delivering the goods — reference to song by Judas Priest released in 1978. Page 88.

ECG - An electrocardiogram is a test that can be used to check your heart's rhythm and electrical activity. Pages 21, 73, 95, 96 & 101.

Elvis with his suspicious mind may suspect foul play – reference to Elvis Presley's recording of suspicious minds. Page 177.

Go walkabout – to wander around from place to place in a protracted or leisurely way. Page 33.

Groundhog Day – 1993 comedy film starring Bill Murray. Page 99.

Hannibal Lector – fictional character in the novels by Thomas Harris, portrayed by Anthony Hopkins in the film 'The Silence of the Lambs.' Page 29.

Hulk Hogan – American professional wrestler. Page 178.

It is just like being in 'The A-Team,' and I love it when a plan comes together – reference to the American action-adventure TV series that ran on NBC from 1983 to 1987 about former members of a fictitious United States Army Special Forces unit. Page 180.

I'm coming home I've done my time – reference to Tony Orlando and Dawn's 1973 recording of the song 'Tie a Yellow Ribbon round the old oak tree.' Page 56.

Indiana Jones – series of action, adventure films starring Harrison Ford. Page 158.

It was like the worst sort of bush tucker trial and I nearly say. 'I am a participant, get me out of here.' – reference to TV program 'I'm a celebrity.' Page 87.

Jeremy Beadle – host of the practical joke TV program 'Beadles About'. Page 24.

Minotaur - a mythical creature with the head and tail of a bull and the body of a man. Page 67.

Mr Benn – a character created by David McKee who appears in several of his novels and an animated TV series. Page 36.

Paul Daniels – reference to magician and TV presenter Paul Daniels and his catchphrase. Page 121 & 122.

Relief of Mafeking – reference to the siege of Mafeking when the town was surrounded by a Boer force of some 5,000 men lasting for seven months from October 1899. Page 87.

Resus trolley – a trolley which is easily accessible containing a wide range of equipment and drugs which would be needed immediately in an emergency resuscitation situation. Page 48.

Road to Damascus – apostle Paul's conversion to Christianity. Page 76 & 115.

Star ship Enterprise, Captain Kirk, more thrust Scotty – reference to long running NBC TV series 'Star Trek'. Page 35.

Steve Austin – character from the TV series 'The Six Million Dollar Man,' a severely injured test pilot is rebuilt with nuclear-powered bionic limbs. Page 187.

Storming the Bastille - July 1789, a Paris prison known as the Bastille, was attacked by an angry and aggressive mob. Page 131.

The Benny Hill Show – a smutty British comedy TV show starring Benny Hill that aired between 1955 and 1989. Page 54.

The Man in the Iron mask - novel by Alexandre Dumas. Page 29.

The Twilight Zone – 1959 American mystical TV series. Page 52.

They say there are seven wonders in this world, meeting Anna and having the children count as my seven, but I was about to find number eight - reference to the lyrics of the song 'Venus in Blue Jeans' released in 1962 by Jimmy Clanton. Page 13.

This must be how Joseph felt, I think about asking her if we are in Bethlehem not Southmead – reference to the Nativity where there was no room at the Inn. Page 53.

White coat syndrome - high blood pressure that occurs at a doctor's surgery or in a medical setting, but not in other settings. Page 22.

You are Batman and Robin to my Commissioner Gordon – reference to the 1960's TV series where the crime fighting duo would repeatedly come to Commissioner Gordon's rescue.

About the author

I have lived and worked near Bristol all my life, I have known Anna since we were both 15 and we have been married for more than 30 years. This is my first adventure into the world of writing. I believe that GDNF could be a cure for Parkinson's and other Neurological diseases, as such, I know it deserves more research and quickly.

Printed in Great Britain
by Amazon